MEN AND WOMEN IN MEDICAL SCHOOL

How They Change and How They Compare

Jane Leserman

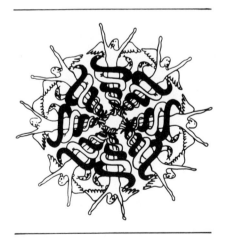

PRAEGER

PRAEGER SPECIAL STUDIES • PRAEGER SCIENTIFIC

Library of Congress Cataloging in Publication Data

Leserman, Jane.
    Men and women in medical school.

    Bibliography: p.
    Includes index.
    1. Medical students—United States—Attitudes—
Longitudinal studies.   2. Women medical students—United States—
Attitudes—Longitudinal studies.   3. Professional
socialization—United States—Sex differences—Longitudinal
studies.   4. Medical education—United States—
Sex differences—Longitudinal studies.   5. Medical
education—Social aspects—United States.   I. Title.
[DNLM: 1. Physician-patient relations.   2. Physicians,
Women—United States.   3. Schools, Medical—United States.
4. Sex characteristics.   W 21 L628m]
R745.L53   610′.7′39   81-7313
ISBN 0-03-058026-9   AACR2

Published in 1981 by Praeger Publishers
CBS Educational and Professional Publishing
A Division of CBS, Inc.
521 Fifth Avenue, New York, New York 10175 U.S.A.

© 1981 by Praeger Publishers

123456789   145   987654321

Printed in the United States of America

2199146

This book is dedicated to my extended family.

You know who you are.

ACKNOWLEDGMENTS

Among the many people who have helped me from the beginning of this research project to the end, two stand out for their enormous contributions. To Jim House and Linda George I express my sincerest gratitude. As chair of my dissertation committee at Duke University and later as a helpful adviser, Jim House has been extremely supportive, encouraging, and patient. Jim has mastered the fine art of giving instructive criticism. His excellent criticisms and insightful suggestions have taught me how to express and organize my ideas more clearly and succinctly. There is no way I can thank him enough for all the time he has spent poring over drafts of my work. One of the reasons I originally chose Jim for the chair of my dissertation committee was because of his fondness for pigs. I figured that anybody who likes pigs must be a compassionate and kind person. My intuition proved correct; I could not have made a better choice.

I will always be grateful to Linda George for all the time she has spent consulting on statistical questions, reviewing this manuscript, and giving emotional support. This book could not have been written without someone like Linda—someone I could call on (and did call on many times) to answer numerous statistical, stylistic, and substantive questions. Her sensible advice, emotional support, and incredible patience always made me feel less anxious about writing this book. Linda's critiques and willingness to help, despite her own busy schedule, were indispensable. As a friend and adviser, Linda has gone far beyond the call of duty.

Two other patient readers of this book, Carol Weisman and Pat Rieker, also deserve a warm note of thanks. Each took the time to carefully read sections of this manuscript and give their thoughtful criticisms. This book has been much improved by following their suggestions and advice.

I also want to express my gratitude to the following people for their technical, administrative, and other assistance that furthered the progress of my research: Babe Andrew, Ann Bell, Dick Campbell, Dick Landerman, Grace Madison, Jim O'Reilly, Shirley Osterhout, Louise Rochelle, and Robert Wilson.

I feel extremely lucky to have had Becky Taylor, my friend and colleague, do the typing for this manuscript. Her accuracy and speed as a typist, her advanced education in the field of sociology, and her warmth as a friend made her the perfect person for the job. Becky, as well as Marni Goldshlag and Roger Madison, assisted with the proofreading of the manuscript. Many thanks to them for their editorial suggestions and for helping with the tedious aspects of book writing. My appreciation also to Marni Goldshlag, Steve Beatrous, and Carol Stack for their title suggestions.

For their continuous emotional support, encouragement, and intellectual stimulation I would also like to thank my husband Roger, my family (Lucille, Milton, Robert, Alma, and Curlee), and my friends (Bigfoot, Didi, Judy, Kris, Marni, Patti, Randee, Sandy, Steve, and Susan). To all of them I give a collective hug.

Last, but not least, I wish to express my appreciation to the medical students in North Carolina who so willingly participated in this study. Without their cooperation this research would not have been possible.

CONTENTS

LIST OF TABLES AND FIGURES

INTRODUCTION

Initially, I became interested in studying medical students for two reasons. I was overwhelmed with the numerous problems that beset modern medicine, and I wondered if medical students would hold values that further aggravated this situation. It seemed that medical educators were doing little to address such problems as physician maldistribution, the depersonalization of care, the accelerating costs of health care, and discrimination toward minority patients and physicians. Since improvement in the delivery and quality of medical care will depend in part on future doctors' greater awareness of and concern about these problems, I decided to study how medical students' values concerning current health issues change from their first to last year of medical school. If medical education results in students adopting values that aggravate current health-care problems, then medical school administrators need to reevaluate their institutions' dominant values and priorities.

A second reason for studying medical students was the presence for the first time in the United States of more than a token number of women in medical school. In 1970 only 11.1 percent of freshman medical school students nationwide were women compared with 23.8 percent in 1975 when this study was initiated.[1] Women medical students have been neglected in most previous studies of medical education so that including men and women in an updated sequel to the famous investigations Boys in White[2] and The Student-Physician[3] is not only feasible now but is greatly needed. Existing research on women medical students and physicians has focused primarily on the problems women face in a male profession and in balancing career and family commitments. Thus, this book reports one of the first major longitudinal studies comparing the professional orientations of women and men in medical school.

The recent increase in the proportion of women in medical school raises the question of how the presence of women will affect the practice and profession of medicine. If women hold different values and choose different types of medical careers than men, the influx of women in medicine may have implications for health-care delivery and quality. We might expect women to be more humanitarian and egalitarian in relating to patients than men; the traditional feminine role emphasizes empathy and nurturance, whereas the traditional masculine role is linked with aggressiveness and dominance. Furthermore, the women's movement may have a politicizing effect on women contributing to their social concern and sensitivity to discrimination toward minorities in medicine.

At a recent conference on women in medicine, one participant cautioned that there has been a

> prior assumption that if we increase the number of women in medicine this will have a . . . beneficial effect on the health care of women and men, and . . . improve the quality of the health care provided by women physicians and by men physicians. But we do not actually know that this is going to happen. [4]

One of the main goals of this book is to describe differences in the professional values and expectations of male and female medical students in order to evaluate whether women will have a beneficial impact on health care.

To compare the professional orientations of male and female medical students and to assess how these orientations change during training, questionnaire data were collected from all freshman medical students in North Carolina in 1975 and again during their senior year. Although a small number of interviews with medical students were also conducted, most of this book will focus on the analysis of questionnaire data.

The book then addresses the following research questions, which summarize its major themes:

1. What are medical students' professional orientations upon entrance to medical school?
2. How and why do these orientations change from their freshman year to their senior year?
3. How and why do the professional orientations of men and women medical students differ upon entrance to medical school?
4. Does medical education affect men's and women's orientations differently, and if so, why?

Some of the issues raised in the first two questions are covered in Chapter 5. A discussion of the implications of these orientation changes for medical education and health care is included in the same chapter.

After delineating the professional orientation changes that occur during medical school, the question of why these changes may have resulted is examined in Chapter 6. Multivariate statistical techniques are utilized to test proposed explanations for the findings.

Chapter 7 presents differences in the professional orientations of men and women in their first and last years of medical school. The author addresses not only orientation differences that exist between the sexes upon entrance to school, but also whether four years of training tends to obscure these variations. The implications for medical education, health care, and the medical profession of sex differences in professional orientation are also discussed.

Chapter 8 examines why the orientations of men and women differ upon entering school and why over time the sexes change uniquely on some orientations. Whereas Chapter 7 reports findings that are mainly descriptive, Chapter 8 presents a multivariate analysis explaining sex differences in professional orientations initially and the differential socialization of men and women.

The professional orientations under investigation concern values and expectations relevant to current problems with the delivery and quality of health care. These include the dehumanizing and authoritarian way that physicians relate to patients, the need to change the political and economic organization of the medical profession, the prejudicial treatment toward women physicians and patients, and the geographic and specialty maldistribution of physicians. Although many other problems have been enumerated by critics of the profession, this book will focus on these four problem areas. Further specification and rationale for the selection of professional values will be presented in Chapter 1.

Chapter 2 presents a review of the literature concerning socialization in medical school and sex differences in the orientation of men and women in medicine. The results of previous medical student and physician studies are reported and the chapter concludes with the findings anticipated in this book.

Chapter 3 includes a discussion of data collection techniques and the measurement of important variables. Descriptions of the students' backgrounds and some initial comparisons among the schools are presented in Chapter 4. Finally, a summary of the findings, a discussion of their implications, and some policy recommendations are presented in the concluding chapter.

If values have significance for actual medical practice, then the findings regarding the research questions addressed in this book may have major implications for medical schools, the medical profession, and health care. If, for example, students become less concerned with the needs of patients as they go through training, one must ask whether medical education is contributing to health-care problems. This book also addresses the issue of what the recent influx of women in medicine will mean for medical education, the medical profession, and medical practice.

NOTES

1. "Undergraduate Medical Education," Journal of the American Medical Association 243 (March 1980): 853.

2. Howard S. Becker, Blanche Geer, Everette C. Hughes, and Anselm L. Strauss, Boys in White (Chicago: University of Chicago Press, 1961).

3. Robert K. Merton, George G. Reader, and Patricia L. Kendall, eds., The Student-Physician: Introductory Studies in the Sociology of Medical Education (Cambridge, Mass.: Harvard University Press, 1957).

4. John Walsh, "Summary of the Conference," in Women in Medicine 1976, ed. Carolyn Spieler (New York: Josiah Macy, Jr. Foundation, 1977), p. 78.

1

PROFESSIONAL VALUES
AND EXPECTATIONS

One aim of medical school is to transform students into physicians. During this educational experience the medical student is bombarded with new knowledge, skills, values, and perspectives. The acquisition of these has been labeled professional socialization. Since this research focuses on how students' orientations change during this intense period of acculturation, the concept of professional values as used in this study and in previous research must be clarified before addressing how socialization affects these values. To begin the discussion of professional values, the author's theoretical perspective is explained so that the selection and interpretation of values can be better understood.

THEORETICAL PERSPECTIVE

In the field of medicine, professional values may refer to a wide variety of attitudes and opinions concerning the profession and the practice of medicine. The numerous authors studying medical students and physicians focus on a large range of professional values.[1] These authors either subtly or overtly imply a theoretical bias indicated by their choice and interpretation of values studied. The adoption of particular values by medical students can be viewed as instrumental, detrimental, or irrelevant to the delivery of good health care. An author's interpretation of professional values is part of his or her broader perspective on professions, in this case the medical profession.

There are two main perspectives on the role of the medical profession in society that can be thought of as two ends of a continuum. These approaches will be labeled conflict and functionalist, labels that have been used in other contexts, most commonly in differentiating

1

theories of stratification and the function of classes in society. Conflict theorists focus on the inherent conflict between the interests of powerful groups (such as the organizations that represent the medical profession) and the interests of the public.[2] The functionalist label has been applied to theories that view such institutions as the medical profession as primarily concerned with meeting the collective goals of the larger society.[3] These labels are somewhat confusing, since we can conceptualize both perspectives in terms of the question, Functional for whom or what? Conflict theorists view the organization of the medical profession as functional for the maintenance of professional autonomy; that is, an occupation's control over its own work, who can perform the tasks and services, the methods and content of performing a task, the knowledge base, and its relationships with certain other occupations. The functionalists, on the other hand, tend to focus on the organization's positive consequences or functions for the larger society so that they often assume if a system operates there must be satisfactory outcomes. Whereas functionalists view autonomy as necessary for the good performance of a profession, conflict theorists view professional autonomy as an end in itself.

The functions of professional values can also be interpreted within the framework of one's particular theoretical bias. To the conflict theorist, values and norms of the profession are aimed at maintaining and legitimating professional autonomy, so that many so-called service values are viewed as rationalizations that sanction professional self-regulation, privilege, and license. Furthermore, to achieve autonomy, professions are viewed as fostering the belief that not only is the group competent in its professed skill and knowledge but also that the knowledge is difficult and beyond the understanding of the general public. Thus conflict theorists see that professionals often mystify their knowledge, that is, emphasize the difference between professional and lay knowledge in order to claim a monopoly on its use. Physicians' use of jargon with patients and their emphasis on the "objective," "technical," and "scientific" quality of their knowledge are typical ways that physicians often mystify the public. Recognizing the tendency of professionals in medicine to mystify their knowledge, one author states that professionalism "tends to set apart; tends to isolate and insulate the professional group from the mundane masses; it gathers the cloak of sanctity about itself and criticism becomes a sacrilege."[4] Although conflict theorists do not deny the actual complexity of a profession's specialized knowledge, they emphasize how the successful claim to knowledge and values reinforcing that claim result in the profession's powerful monopoly in society at large and physicians' domination over patients.

Alternatively, the functionalists do not view professional values, such as service ideals and codes of ethics, as mere rationalizations for maintaining power and prestige. Instead, they interpret these values as legitimate attempts by the profession at being responsive to societal needs. Thus, the need to socially control professions is solved by individual adherence to service ideals. Functionalists claim that professionals are more altruistic than people in business; however, most of these theorists admit that this is an ideal characteristic of professionals that may not reflect reality. Parsons specifies that the service orientation is not meant to refer to individual motives but to the character of a profession. [5] Conflict theorists, to the contrary, interpret such actions as limiting the number of doctors and opposing most national health insurance plans as resembling the actions of a union rather than an institution oriented to service.

Thus, choosing which professional values to study and interpreting these selected values are based on a researcher's theoretical perspective. In conceptualizing and carrying out the research project reported here, the author has assumed a conflict perspective. Therefore, the author focuses on values and expectations relevant to health-care problems, those being the points of conflict between professional and public interests. Many values endorsed by physicians and the medical profession are therefore considered detrimental to the delivery and quality of health care in this country. For example, due to the shortage of primary-care physicians it is in the public interest for medical students not to specialize. [6] Students, however, experience pressure and encouragement in medical school to specialize, owing in part to the high income and status of most specialists and the security in knowing a smaller body of knowledge.

Further specification of the values under investigation will be presented later in this chapter. A discussion will follow of the way specific professional values have been selected and interpreted in previous research.

PREVIOUS RESEARCH

Although there have been numerous studies of medical students' values, most previous measures of professional orientation lack comparability, specificity, reliability, and relevance to health-care issues. The rationale for selection of particular values in these studies is rarely stated, most studies analyzing responses to a wide variety of single-item questions. The lack of theoretical justification for the inclusion of variables and the reliance on only one item to measure a concept leads to questioning the health-care relevance and the reliability of these professional value measures. It is best to have indexes or scales composed of at least a few items tapping each concept, since these are less affected by measurement error than single items.

Studies of medical students have often focused on vague concepts, such as idealism and cynicism, that can only be assumed to indicate students' potential treatment of and attitudes toward patients. These vague concepts are used rather differently in medical student studies, making comparisons of the findings somewhat difficult. Becker and his colleagues measure idealism in terms of medical students' desire to help people, lack of interest in money, belief that medical skills and knowledge are necessary for success, and belief that medicine is the best of all professions. [7] In contrast, Eron defines cynicism as an attitude toward human nature (for example, "most people would lie to get ahead") and not as a view concerning medical practice. [8]

Many questions often asked in studies of medical students and physicians elicit idealistic and socially acceptable responses and therefore are not particularly informative. For example, studies often ask some variant to the question, "How important in your choice of medicine is helping people or making a large income?"[9] From these measures authors often conclude that students are altruistic without probing any deeper into students' motivations or personal ambitions. Since there is little questioning of the functionalist assumption that professionals are inclined toward public service as opposed to personal ambition, responses to these questions that elicit socially acceptable answers are taken at face value. Furthermore, it is unclear what implications, if any, responses to such measures as idealism, cynicism, or those prompting socially acceptable replies will have for patient care.

The papers based on the famous panel study reported in The Student-Physician tend to focus on more specific values related to the doctor/patient relationship. [10] Values include the importance of social and emotional factors in illness, preference for patients with physical illness, and the tendency to view patients as disease entities. The reliance on one questionnaire item to measure each of these values makes the reliability of these professional value measures problematic. In addition, the authors adopt the viewpoint of the medical school faculty so that values defined as appropriate by the faculty are assumed to be good for medical practice. The functionalist interpretation of values leaves little room for a critical evaluation of the orientations learned in medical school.

In addition to the research already mentioned, many studies administer to medical students value scales that have been prepared for numerous educated populations. [11] These include such inventories as the Allport, Vernon, and Lindzey Study of Values[12] and Gordon's Survey of Interpersonal Values. [13] Since the scales in these inventories are designed to measure fairly general values and personality constructs, one must question their relevance when given to medical student populations. For example, on the Allport, Vernon, and Lindzey scale of social concern, respondents are asked their opinion on the importance of human rights and social welfare in society and their personal preference for helping others, but are not asked questions specific to social concern in medicine. It is certainly conceivable that students might favor social welfare but not approve of socialized medicine. Furthermore, many of the items on these inventories are somewhat dated because they were developed decades ago.

PROFESSIONAL VALUES AND EXPECTATIONS

When undertaking the present study, the author was faced with the challenging problem of developing reliable, valid, and meaningful measures of professional orientation. In contrast to previous research, specific professional values regarding the practice of medicine and the structure of the medical profession have been selected for examination in this study. The rationale for selection of values and expectations rests on their relevance to health-care problems, particularly values and conditions for which physicians and the profession have been most criticized.

Values and expectations pertaining to health-care problems have been selected in order to ascertain some of the health-care implications of professional socialization. In other words, we can determine if students become more or less committed to values and careers aimed at relieving health-care problems during their medical training. Speculations can also be made on the potential health-care effects of the recent increase in women physicians by determining sex differences on these health-related values.

Rather than just measuring vague constructs, this research focuses on a range of more specific values. For example, instead of assuming that a cynical world view implies cynical attitudes toward patients, specific values pertaining to the doctor/patient relationship are included. It is hoped that describing medical students' specific health-care-related orientations will provide a more realistic picture of students upon entrance to and departure from medical school than previous research, which measured idealistic responses. Some general measures have also been included in this study (such as how important helping people, income, and status are in career selection) in order to facilitate comparisons with previous research. In addition, most measures of values consist of two or more correlated questionnaire items so that these variables are more reliable than previous single-item measures.

The values and expectations chosen for this study in no way comprise a definitive list and their significance for health care is certainly subject to other interpretations than those presented by the

FIGURE 1.1

Professional Values and Expectations Organized by Health-Care
Problem Areas

I. Physicians' Relationships with Patients
   1. The importance of physicians providing health information
      concerning diagnosis and treatment to patients, including
      patients having access to their own medical records.
   2. The freedom of patients and other doctors to be critical of
      physicians; that is, patients not having absolute confidence in
      physicians' judgments and physicians making public criticisms
      of their colleagues.
   3. Social and psychological factors, including empathy and rap-
      port, are considered important aspects of health care.
   4. Helping people is seen as an important part of one's medical
      career.

II. Political and Economic Change in the Profession
   1. Favor reduction in the profession's control over health care
      through government intervention and socialized medicine.
   2. Favor a National Service Corps for physicians so that physi-
      cians would have to serve in a medically deprived area.
   3. Favor changing the health-care system so that profits are not
      made from health care.
   4. Favor reduction in physicians' status and income.
   5. High status and income are seen as an important part of one's
      medical career.
   6. Intending to work for political and social change in medicine.
   7. Intending to do volunteer work as a physician.

III. The Treatment of Women Physicians and Patients
   1. Awareness of the profession's and the public's discrimination
      against women doctors.
   2. Acknowledging the pressure on women physicians to choose
      certain fields like pediatrics and to avoid specialties like
      surgery.
   3. Favoring an increase in the number of women physicians.
   4. Acknowledging the patronizing and insensitive treatment of
      female patients by physicians.

IV. Physician Maldistribution
   1. Expecting to practice primary-care medicine.
   2. Expecting to practice in a rural area.
   3. Expecting to practice in an inner-city ghetto area.
   4. Committed to choosing a specialty and geographic area that
      needs physicians.

author. Many values are omitted, such as those pertaining directly to technical competence, although these, too, are important in the delivery of quality medical care. Nevertheless, because many previous research conceptions of professional values have lacked comparability, specificity, reliability, and relevance to health care, this study contributes theoretically and methodologically to the clarification and measurement of professional orientations.

The professional orientations under investigation concern four health-care problem areas:

1. Physicians' relationships with patients; the need to humanize doctor/patient interactions and involve patients in health-care decisions;

2. Political and economic organization of the medical profession; that is, the importance of reducing the profession's excessive control over health care and physicians' income and status;

3. The prejudicial treatment of women physicians and patients and the underrepresentation of women in medicine;

4. Geographic and specialty maldistribution of physicians; that is, the need for doctors in rural and inner-city ghetto areas and in primary-care medicine.

The specific values and expectations pertaining to these four problem areas analyzed in this study are listed in Figure 1.1. The discussion that follows presents literature critical of the country's health-care system in order to show that the professional orientations under investigation are relevant to current health-care problems. Furthermore, the potential implications for health care of students advocating views and planning careers consistent with remedying these problems are also discussed. No attempt is made to discuss all the problems that plague our health system today since that would go beyond the scope of this book.

Physicians' Relationships with Patients

Physicians, the medical profession, and medical schools have long been criticized for their lack of attention to the problems of humanizing doctor/patient interactions; that is, learning how to treat the patient as a person and not as a disease entity. [14] Included in this critique is the need to improve doctor/patient communication by reducing physician dominance and mystique and to consider the social and psychological aspects of patient care and not just the physical dimensions. Values that accentuate the difference between lay and professional knowledge are considered tactics that perpetuate physician dominance and mystique. In this study, values that may aid in creating more egalitarian and humane doctor/patient interactions are considered beneficial for the quality of health care.

The following specific professional values are aimed at reducing physician authority and mystique: the importance of physicians providing health information to patients concerning diagnosis and treatment, including patients having access to their own medical records; and being critical of physicians, that is, patients not having absolute confidence in physicians' judgments and physicians making public criticisms of their colleagues.

Research shows that both physicians and patients enter into a professional relationship expecting it to be vastly unequal. To medical students and physicians the ideal physician is dominant, strong-willed, and rigid, whereas the ideal patient is compliant, weak-willed, stoic, and uncomplaining.[15] When hospital patients have been asked what physicians expect of them, most indicate trust, cooperation, and confidence; moreover, many fear that not conforming to these expectations will result in inadequate care.[16] These fears seem justified since some studies have indicated that physicians admit to giving better medical care to people who fit the ideal patient image than those who are less stoic and less cooperative.[17]

Patient dependence on physicians is further strengthened by the belief that the doctor knows best, because physicians have asserted that clients are not competent to evaluate professionals' work or to understand their own medical problems.[18] Therefore, physicians tend not to give health information to patients and tend to expect absolute confidence from patients. Interestingly, welfare recipients' evaluations of physicians are consistent with professional criteria for assessing physician performance.[19] Thus, supposedly ignorant clients are able to make accurate evaluations, although medical professionals tend to deny this. Control over information may be used by doctors to maintain their dominance while keeping patients dependent.

As well as expecting patients to be uncritical, physicians disapprove of colleague criticism in front of patients.[20] Public censure would call into question physicians' authority and claims to expertise. Physicians are therefore reluctant to testify against each other in malpractice suits for fear of destroying some of the mystique surrounding their claims to knowledge.

Empirical evidence shows that both withholding information and expecting absolute confidence from patients may have negative consequences for medical care. Authoritarian physicians who do little to communicate with patients are likely to find that their patients do not comply with medical orders, thereby reducing the effectiveness of the treatments.[21] Furthermore, physicians and medical students who will not admit to their own limitations and emphasize the need for patient confidence in physicians have been ranked lower in clinical performance by their colleagues.[22] Thus excessive assertion of physicians' authority appears detrimental to physicians' clinical performance.

Physicians' relationships with patients have been extremely paternalistic since, traditionally, doctors have been solely responsible for determining patients' needs. In 1972, however, the American Hospital Association issued a patients' bill of rights giving patients the right to obtain from their doctors complete information concerning their diagnosis, treatment, and prognosis in terms that the patient can understand. Although only hospitals that adopt this bill of rights are bound by it, this document is a first step in transferring health-care responsibility back to the patient.

Recently, an increasing number of people have been demanding greater equality in the doctor/patient relationship. The holistic health movement now gaining momentum in this country has focused on taking responsibility for one's own health care rather than total dependence on and trust in physicians. People are beginning to realize that relying totally on physicians' advice has resulted in unnecessary surgery, overmedication, and iatrogenic disorders (illness or harm caused by physician intervention). Although patients may pay a high price if they do not conform to physicians' expectations, they may also pay a high price if they do so blindly: deformed babies from mothers taking thalidomide, pelvic inflamatory disease from the Dalkon Shield (an interuterine device to prevent pregnancy), and cervical and vaginal cancer in the daughters of women who took DES (diethylstilbestrol) during pregnancy.*

For many years physicians have been criticized for ignoring the social and psychological aspects of health care including establishing rapport with clients.[23] The problem starts in medical school where there is an emphasis on learning technical skills and treating diseases rather than on learning interpersonal skills and treating the whole patient by taking into account social and emotional factors. Al-

---

*There are different points of view on the importance ascribed to trusting totally in one's doctor. The placebo effect may not work if patients do not have absolute faith in their physicians. There is certainly more than a grain of truth in the expression that "the doctor himself is his best medicine." If patients become more critical of physicians, placebo medicine may no longer bring dramatic cures; however, a new sense of control over one's own health care may have a similar healing effect. Relaxation, attainable in many ways besides through blind faith, may be the most important healing agent.

though it is simpler and quicker to treat physical symptoms as opposed to emotional problems, there appears to be a strong link between the two. Recent research suggests that a wide variety of physical ailments are correlated with life stress.[24] Therefore, it seems that a comprehensive medical approach would take into account both the physical and psychological factors in health care.

In addition, doctor/patient rapport appears to affect patient care directly because compliance with doctors' advice is linked to friendly doctor/patient relationships.[25] Skillful clinical performance, as judged by physicians, has also been associated with physicians who are nurturant and who pay attention to patients' emotional health.[26] Interpersonal skills can contribute to the diagnosis of disease problems.

Values of humanizing doctor/patient interaction have been included in this research because they directly address important health-care problems. More comprehensive and egalitarian health care will depend in part on the extent to which future doctors give health information to clients, do not demand absolute confidence from patients, accept public criticism of colleagues, and pay attention to the social and psychological needs of their patients.

Political and Economic Change
in the Medical Profession

After reviewing studies of medical student attitudes, one author states, "It is noteworthy that very little work has been done in the effort to identify tendencies toward liberalism-conservatism in the education of physicians in spite of the continuing and increasing public interest in precisely such questions. . . . The growing interest of the public in the economics of medicine, in its professional organization, and in its participation in political processes is not yet reflected in attitude studies of medical students and doctors."[27] The present study does examine medical students' views on timely issues concerning political and economic change in the organization of the medical profession and the health-care system because these issues address problems in health care today.

Of special interest in this study are controversial issues concerning the reduction in both the medical profession's control over health care and physicians' status and income and the need to change the capitalist organization of the health-care system. A functionalist would interpret the present economic and political organization of medicine as necessary for the smooth functioning of the profession. But professional self-regulation, health care for profit, and large incomes and prestige for physicians are interpreted by this author and many others as contrary to public interest.[28]

The medical profession's almost complete control over its own work leaves little room for public accountability. Because the priorities of this professional monopoly (for example, profits and technical skills) sometimes conflict with the public demand for accessible quality medical care, self-regulation ensures that the profession's interests will come first. Specifically, self-regulation exacerbates such problems as physician maldistribution, rising medical costs, and inadequate quality control because it is not in the interests of physicians to increase the number of doctors, to locate practitioners in areas of need, to lower medical charges, or to have public committees review doctors' work. Furthermore, even problems associated with the doctor/patient relationship are not likely to improve in a monopoly system with little public accountability or outside input into such things as medical curricula.

Government intervention in health care is frowned upon by the medical profession, despite the fact that the government helps to subsidize medical education and medical research. The American Medical Association (AMA)—a union-like organization—led the opposition to Medicare and Medicaid[29] and continues today to oppose national health insurance legislation (except its own plan, which minimizes the government's role in medical care). Although initially the AMA fought against passage of Medicaid and Medicare, these programs have made many doctors rich and have helped to inflate the cost of medical care for the consumer. Government intervention will not necessarily be a panacea for health-care problems because the government often acts in the interests of the medical profession. But government intervention in health care, if done in response to consumer interests, has the potential for improving physician distribution by providing incentives to doctors to locate in need areas; reducing medical costs to patients via a system of socialized medicine, reviewing physicians' fees, or a national health insurance plan; and improving quality control with consumer review boards in addition to peer review.

Besides government programs to decrease medical costs, directly lowering physicians' prestige and income would help curb rising medical charges and also aid in reducing the status differences between practitioners and the public. Therefore, medical students in this study are asked their view toward lowering physicians' status and financial rewards. Previous studies cited before have asked medical students to evaluate the importance of income and status in choosing their career. Because denying personal interest in these rewards is the socially acceptable response for future doctors, the present study also asks students their opinion on lowering physicians' incomes and status. This less personal question is expected to elicit more candid responses.

This study focuses on students' views toward government intervention, the profit system, and lowering physicians' incomes and status in order to see whether our future doctors will be part of the solution or part of the problem. Much more than just liberal doctors are needed for change in the organization of the medical profession, but that could be a contributing factor. Supporting these political and economic reforms in medicine may translate in practice to working in free clinics and charging lower fees.

In addition to values concerning political and economic change in the profession, students' intentions to work for political and social change in medicine are of interest in this study. It is one thing to support liberal causes, but it is another to work for implementing these ideals. Professionals generally have an individualistic orientation to service; that is, they work for particular clients, often in a fee-for-service system, and feel no obligation to serve the public. Therefore medical students may have a vague desire to help people on an individual basis, but they may not express a commitment to social or political service (that is, working to change the medical system so that it is more responsive to public needs). Wanting to help individual patients does not necessarily translate into working for free helath clinics or for improved access to health care for everyone.

Hence, if students intend to work for political and social change in medicine, including volunteer service, and tend to support political and economic change in the medical profession, they may have a limited but beneficial impact on health care. Asking medical students to respond to specific political and economic issues concerning problems in medicine is expected to be more informative than just determining their general political leanings or asking questions that elicit idealistic or socially acceptable values.

Prejudice against Women Physicians and Patients

Discrimination toward women physicians today has its roots in history. Originally the medical schools and medical societies banned women from medicine so that if women wanted to practice they could try to "pass" by dressing like men. Although the first woman was admitted to a U.S. medical school in 1847, it was not until 1879 that many medical schools officially opened their doors to women and not until 1915 that the AMA admitted women to membership in that organization.[30] When women were finally admitted into the medical profession they were not allowed to examine male patients below the waist, although there was no similar prohibition on male physicians in treating women patients. In 1974 a female intern at the University of Michigan was banned from an examination where a man's genitals were exposed, yet her husband, also an intern, was doing pelvic ex-

aminations.[31] Many such historical examples of discrimination toward
women physicians are still occurring.

Discrimination toward women patients today reflects the helpless, subservient view of women in history. Medical theories of the
mid- to late 1880s reinforced and justified the belief that women, especially those in the upper class, were innately weak and defective.
These theories traced female illness to sexual, athletic, or mental
activity so that sex, dancing, reading too much, or ambition could
lead to sickness.[32] Physicians back then helped to keep women dependent, ignorant, homebound, and asexual. Today, women patients
still complain about the patronizing attitudes of male physicians. Furthermore, it was accepted medical practice until the early 1900s to
perform sexual surgery (removal of the clitoris or ovaries) on women
who were accused by parents or husbands of masturbating or unruly
behavior and on those suffering from psychological disorders.[33] Today, hysterectomies (removal of the uterus) are commonly performed
on women for supposed medical reasons, but studies have claimed
that these are often unnecessary because about one-third involve the
removal of normal organs.[34] A glimpse back to the past can help us
understand the origins of present problems experienced by women
physicians and patients.

The increasing number of female physicians and the women's
health movement have fostered greater public awareness of discrimination toward women physicians and patients. Since sexism is a current problem in the health-care system, discrimination toward women
physicians and patients has been a major focus of this research. *
Specifically of interest are orientations acknowledging discrimination
toward women physicians from professionals and the public, the pressure on women physicians to choose particular specialties such as
pediatrics and the pressure not to select fields like surgery, the need
for more women doctors in this country, and the patronizing and insensitive treatment of women patients by physicians.

Frequently mentioned discriminatory practices toward female
medical students and physicians by their medical colleagues include
overt hostility, sexist remarks and jokes, little encouragement or
support, and exclusion of females from discussions and advancement
due in part to the "men's club" atmosphere. The following cite ex-

---

*Although discrimination against black physicians and patients is
also a problem, these issues have not been included in the questionnaire. Certainly racial discrimination affects the quality of health
care, but due to the excessive length of the questionnaire these issues
have been omitted. Since sex differences are the major focus of this
study, questions on sex discrimination were considered more relevant.

amples of discriminatory remarks made by male physicians toward women medical students: "Because of you a man probably went into chiropractic school"; "Why would a girl go into medicine?"; "A woman doesn't belong in the OR [operating room] except as a nurse"; and "Most women don't practice."[35] More subtle examples of discrimination occur during group discussions with faculty where women's comments are ignored, and professors address only the male students or ask only males to do procedures. The examples of prejudice are too numerous to detail here, although recent reports suggest that at least overt discrimination has become less common. The problems for women today revolve around what has been labeled a "discriminatory environment" in medical school that affects women's careers and specialty choices. This includes the subtle forms of discrimination like acts of omission, the devaluing of female traits like sensitivity, and the conflicts between family and career because the time for intense career building occurs simultaneously with the optimal age for having a family.[36]

In addition to discrimination from colleagues and medical school faculty, in the past women in medicine have been subjected to prejudicial attitudes from patients.[37] This is probably less true today as women become more numerous in medicine.

One bias that is cited often is the pressure on women in medicine to choose traditionally female specialties like pediatrics and psychiatry and to avoid male fields like surgery.[38] Among a national sample of recent medical school graduates 17.8 percent of the women plan a pediatric specialty compared with only 7.0 percent of the men, whereas only 6.9 percent of the women intend to select surgery compared with 16.7 percent of the men. Furthermore, from 1960 to 1978 the percentage of women selecting surgery remained stable, whereas the percentage in pediatrics declined somewhat.[39] It seems that women are feeling less pressure to choose pediatrics than two decades ago, but that surgery is still taboo.

The subtle and overt specialization discrimination comes from parents, relatives, and peers as well as medical school faculty. At one medical school, women were less likely to plan a specialty in surgery after their surgery clerkship than before this rotation, whereas the men remained stable in their specialization choice.[40] Apparently females received negative feedback from their peers and instructors about going into surgery, although that clerkship had been considered better than most with regard to discrimination. In surgery, the message to women has been to stay out. In another study, one chief resident reportedly told the women medical students assigned to his rotation, "I don't like women in orthopedics. If you go to the library for the next 2 weeks you can have C's."[41] Under these conditions women tend to choose fields where they will be accepted and where they will not have to fight for approval.

The underrepresentation of women in medicine is another problem facing the profession, because the number of women in medical school has only recently increased. Of the total physicians in the United States in 1977, only 11.2 percent were women.[42] It is the author's belief that in order to improve the treatment of women patients and to ensure the representation of women's interests in research, we will need more women in medicine. Medical schools will have to actively recruit and accept female applicants if the underrepresentation of women physicians is going to be remedied.

Physicians' discriminatory treatment of women patients is another frequently cited problem that has been shown to have its roots in history. Some of the complaints lodged against the medical profession concerning the treatment of women patients include the physicians' lack of sensitivity to and respect for women, an inaccurate view of female sexuality, tendencies to diagnose women's illnesses as psychosomatic, and numerous sexist attitudes.[43] In a recent study of doctor/patient interactions, doctors responded in a less technical way to their female patients than to their male clients even when the questions asked were equally technical. Furthermore, doctors were more likely to see the illnesses of females as psychologically caused than those of males.[44]

In recent gynecology textbooks, women have been portrayed as helpless and childlike, fulfilled only by being mothers. Their physical symptoms (like painful intercourse or painful menstruation) are reduced to emotional causes even though there is empirical evidence to the contrary. Furthermore, recent textbooks ignore well-documented sex research and thus perpetuate myths about female sexuality, such as vaginal orgasm being the only mature response and women being sexually passive and interested in sex only for procreation.[45]

If women accept the passive role perpetuated by doctors' patronizing treatment, then they will be vulnerable to such malpractices as the misdiagnosis of physical illness as solely emotional in nature, unnecessary surgery, the administration of unproved drugs, and subjection to myths and misinformation about their sexual response. The recent self-help movement among women to learn more about women's health care, including self-examination, has been their response to such malpractices and to physicians' neglect of their role as patient educators. Awareness concerning these abuses of women physicians and patients is the first step in solving these problems. If medical students are aware of and sensitive to these issues maybe there will be less sex discrimination in medicine in the future.

Physician Maldistribution

Specialty and geographic maldistribution of physicians are other critical health problems facing us today. There is a shortage of doctors in inner-city and rural areas and in primary-care practice.[46] Primary care refers to physicians of first contact offering a relatively full scope of services and includes family practitioners, pediatricians, internal medicine specialists, and some gynecologists who do little or no surgery.

Contrary to numerous assessments, one recent study suggests that there is no shortage of primary-care physicians since specialists serve as principal care providers for many Americans.[47] This study probably overestimates the amount of primary-care problems that are handled by specialists because it has not taken into account the comprehensiveness of the care offered by specialists, only the continuity of care provided. It seems financially and medically unwise to have specialists provide primary-care services because specialists tend to charge higher fees and have less training in dealing with the larger context of medical ills. If specialists are performing primary-care tasks, it probably indicates a shortage of primary-care doctors more than the ability of specialists to provide these general services and the desirability of having them do so.

Recently, however, there has been some controversy concerning the future shortage of primary-care physicians because the government predicts an overabundance of all physicians by 1990.[48] With physician overabundance, especially in specialties, it is probably less detrimental to have proportionately more primary-care physicians than specialists. Because specialists tend to receive higher fees and to locate in areas where there is an overabundance of doctors, the trend toward specialization aggravates the already high cost of medical care and the geographic maldistribution of physicians. Furthermore, overspecialization has also been linked with unnecessary surgery because the overabundance of surgeons seems to result in excessive surgery. It seems to be a general rule that the more surgeons there are, the more operations there will be, whether needed or not. The oversupply of physicians does not follow the normal market model of supply and demand; the more surgeons in an area, the higher are their fees.[49] With specialization there is also a tendency to study rare diseases that are considered more interesting than common and chronic problems seen most often in primary-care practices. Because there is little research on many common health problems, patients with these uninteresting afflictions may find that their doctors know less about how to treat their problems than how to treat the rare patient with a complex disease.

There seems to be no shortage in the number of physicians nationwide since the United States has one of the highest physician/population ratios in the world. However, maldistribution of existing services does create a health-care delivery problem. Physicians and health-care services are greatly lacking in rural and inner-city ghetto areas, regions populated by low-income persons and blacks.

One of the reasons that the United States ranks one of the highest among industrial countries in its infant mortality rate is that these rates are extremely high among rural and inner-city populations, groups that receive few maternal health services. Infant mortality rates for other portions of the population are much lower than for the poor, the black, and the underserved. In addition, since blacks and other low-income Americans are more likely to have chronic illnesses and to be disabled, geographic maldistribution aggravates these existing health inequities.[50] Of course, the relationship between income and health is reciprocal so that being unhealthy leads to poverty and being poor contributes to sickness. The point, however, is that the portions of the population with the greatest medical need receive proportionately fewer services.

There are many reasons for the long-term trend away from primary-care, rural, and inner-city ghetto practices. As the complexity and the amount of information in medicine has increased, specialty practice has seemed more feasible than trying to grasp the whole spectrum of medical knowledge. In addition, the reliance and dependence on complex medical technologies has forced doctors into more urban areas where elaborate equipment and information on new developments are available. Since specialists work more regular hours and make more money than generalists, there are economic and life-style incentives for choosing a specialty practice. Doctors have a long history of avoiding areas that serve poor populations because these areas net a lower financial return. Other personal considerations keep doctors out of rural areas, such as wanting the educational and cultural activities available only in cities.

If medical students today show more interest in planning a practice in a specialty and geographic area of patient need than students previously, we should see some improvement in health-care delivery. Little or no commitment through medical training to these need areas will perpetuate the geographic and specialty maldistribution of physicians and the health problems associated with these distribution inequities.

SUMMARY

Values and expectations relevant to current health-care problems have been selected in this study in order to present a more realistic picture of medical students than previous research has and to assess the health-care implications of professional socialization. If students begin medical school with good intentions but lose these during training, we must challenge the values taught in medical school. In addition, if new recruits, such as women, hold different values than men, we can speculate on the effect that the recent increase in women physicians will have on health care.

This chapter has shown how the values and expectations chosen for study have implications for health-care delivery and quality. These selected orientations exemplify some of the intense conflicts between professional and public interests in four health-care problem areas: physicians' relationships with patients, change in the organization of the profession, the treatment of women physicians and patients, and geographic and specialty maldistribution of physicians.

The next chapter will review previous medical student research concerning professional socialization in medical school (the fate of values through training), differences in orientation between males and females, and differential socialization of males and females. From this literature review the author will hypothesize expected changes in professional orientations from medical students' first to last year of training and expected differences between males and females on these orientations over time.

NOTES

1. The following list includes some of the older and more well-known studies of medical students' values: Howard S. Becker, Blanche Geer, Everette C. Hughes, and Anselm L. Strauss, Boys in White (Chicago: University of Chicago Press, 1961); Don Cahalan, Patricia Collette, and Norman A. Hilmar, "Career Interests and Expectations of U.S. Medical Students," Journal of Medical Education 32 (August 1957): 557-63; Leonard Eron, "The Effect of Medical Education on Attitudes: A Follow-up Study," Journal of Medical Education 33, pt. 2 (1958): 25-33; and Robert K. Merton, George G. Reader, and Patricia L. Kendall, eds., The Student-Physician: Introductory Studies in the Sociology of Medical Education (Cambridge, Mass.: Harvard University Press, 1957).

2. The following list includes some examples of authors who take a conflict perspective when discussing the medical profession and the health-care system. Robert R. Alford, Health Care Politics (Chicago: University of Chicago Press, 1975); Eliot Freidson, Profession of Medicine: A Study of the Sociology of Applied Knowledge (New York: Dodd Mead, 1970); and Elliott A. Krause, Power and Illness: The Political Sociology of Health and Medical Care (New York: Elsevier North-Holland, 1977).

3. The following list includes some examples of authors who take a functionalist view of professions. Ernest Greenwood, "Attributes of a Profession," Social Work 2 (July 1957): 44-55; Robert K. Merton, "Some Preliminaries to a Sociology of Medical Education,"

in Student-Physician, ed. Merton, Reader, and Kendall, pp. 3-79; and Talcott Parsons, "The Professions and Social Structure," Social Forces 17 (May 1939): 457-67.

4. Joel B. Montague, Jr., "Medicine and the Concept of Professionalism," Sociological Inquiry 33 (Winter 1963): 47.

5. Parsons, "Professions and Social Structure," pp. 457-67.

6. Charles E. Lewis, Rashi Fein, and David Mechanic, A Right to Health: The Problem of Access to Primary Medical Care (New York: John Wiley & Sons, 1976).

7. Becker et al., Boys in White, pp. 70-79.

8. Eron, "Effect of Medical Education on Attitudes," pp. 25-33.

9. See, for example, Samuel W. Bloom, Power and Dissent in the Medical School (New York: Free Press, 1973), pp. 93-107; and Leonard Reissman, Ralph Platou, S. H. Sledge, and D. H. Malone, "The Motivation and Socialization of Medical Students," Journal of Health and Human Behavior 1 (Fall 1960): 174-82.

10. Merton, Reader, and Kendall, eds., Student-Physician.

11. See, for example, Leonard V. Gordon and Ivan N. Mensh, "Values of Medical School Students at Different Levels of Training," Journal of Educational Psychology 53 (1962): 48-51; Edwin B. Hutchins, "The AAMC Longitudinal Study: Implications for Medical Education," Journal of Medical Education 39 (1964): 265-77; and Isabel R. Juan, Rosalia E. A. Paiva, Harold B. Haley, and Robert O'Keefe, "High and Low Levels of Dogmatism in Relation to Personality Characteristics of Medical Students: A Follow-up Study," Psychological Reports 34 (1974): 303-15.

12. Gordon W. Allport, Philip E. Vernon, and Gardner Lindzey, Study of Values (Boston: Houghton Mifflin, 1960).

13. Leonard V. Gordon, Survey of Interpersonal Values (Chicago: Science Research Associates, 1960).

14. Michael Balint, The Doctor, His Patient and the Illness (New York: International Universities Press, 1957), pp. 11-68; Samuel W. Bloom, "Some Implications of Studies in the Professionalization of the Physician," in Patients, Physicians and Illness, ed. E. Gartley Jaco (Glencoe, Ill.: Free Press, 1958), pp. 313-21; and Steven Jonas, Medical Mystery: The Training of Doctors in the United States (New York: W. W. Norton, 1978), pp. 72-77.

15. Richard Christie and Robert K. Merton, "Procedures for the Sociological Study of the Values Climate of Medical Schools," Journal of Medical Education 33, pt. 2 (October 1958): 125-53; and Judith Lorber, "Good Patients and Problem Patients: Conformity and Deviance in a General Hospital," in Patients, Physicians and Illness, ed. E. Gartley Jaco, 3d ed. (New York: Free Press, 1979), pp. 202-17.

16. Lorber, "Good Patients and Problem Patients," pp. 202-17; Daisy L. Tagliacozzo and Hans O. Mauksch, "The Patient's View of the Patient's Role," in Patients, Physicians and Illness, ed. E. Gartley Jaco, 3d ed. (New York: Free Press, 1979), pp. 185-201.

17. Morris J. Daniels, "Affect and Its Control in the Medical Intern," American Journal of Sociology 66 (November 1960): 259-67; and Irving K. Zola, "Culture and Symptoms—An Analysis of Patients' Presenting Complaints," American Sociological Review 31 (October 1966): 615-30.

18. Freidson, Profession of Medicine, pp. 137-84; and Wilbert E. Moore, The Professions: Roles and Rules (New York: Russell Sage Foundation, 1970), pp. 87-130.

19. Arnold I. Kisch and Leo G. Reeder, "Client Evaluation of Physician Performance," Journal of Health and Social Behavior 10 (March 1969): 51-58.

20. Freidson, Profession of Medicine, pp. 137-84; Moore, The Professions, pp. 109-30; and Merton, "Preliminaries to Sociology of Medical Education, pp. 73-75.

21. Barry Blackwell, "Drug Therapy: Patient Compliance," New England Journal of Medicine 289 (August 1973): 249-52; Milton S. Davis, "Variations in Patients' Compliance with Doctors' Advice: An Empirical Analysis of Patterns of Communication," American Journal of Public Health 58 (February 1968): 274-88; and Vida Francis, Barbara M. Korsch, and Marie J. Morris, "Gaps in Doctor-Patient Communication," New England Journal of Medicine 280 (March 1969): 535-40.

22. Ralph Liske, Robert Ort, and Amasa Ford, "Clinical Performances and Related Traits of Medical Students and Faculty Physicians," Journal of Medical Education 39 (January 1964): 69-80.

23. Balint, The Doctor, His Patient and the Illness, pp. 11-68; Bloom, "Some Implications of Studies in the Professionalization of Physicians," pp. 313-21; and Jonas, Medical Mystery, pp. 72-77.

24. Barbara S. Dohrenwend and Bruce P. Dohrenwend, eds., Stressful Life Events: Their Nature and Effects (New York: John Wiley & Sons, 1974).

25. Blackwell, "Drug Therapy: Patient Compliance," pp. 249-52; Davis, "Variations in Patients' Compliance with Doctors' Advice," pp. 274-88; and Francis, Korsch, and Morris, "Gaps in Doctor-Patient Communication," pp. 235-40.

26. Liske, Ort, and Ford, "Clinical Performance and Related Traits," pp. 69-80.

27. Samuel W. Bloom, "Socialization for the Physician's Role: A Review of Some Contributions of Research to Theory," in Becoming a Physician, ed. Eileen C. Shapiro and Leah M. Lowenstein (Cambridge, Mass.: Ballinger, 1979), pp. 28-29.

28. See, for example, Alford, Health Care Politics, pp. 1-21; Freidson, Profession of Medicine; and Robert S. McCleery, Louise T. Keelty, Mimi Lam, Russell E. Phillips, and Terrence M. Quirin, One Life-One Physician: An Inquiry into the Medical Profession's Performance in Self Regulation (Washington, D.C.: Public Affairs Press, 1971).

29. Richard Harris, A Sacred Trust (New York: New American Library, 1966).

30. Geoffrey Marks and William K. Beatty, Women in White (New York: Charles Scribner's Sons, 1972), pp. 83-115.

31. Gena Corea, The Hidden Malpractice: How American Medicine Mistreats Women (New York: Jove, 1977), p. 31.

32. Barbara Ehrenreich and Deirdre English, Complaints and Disorders: The Sexual Politics of Sickness (Old Westbury, N.Y.: Feminist Press, 1973), pp. 5-44.

33. Ibid., pp. 32-38; and G. J. Barker-Benfield, "Sexual Surgery in Late-Nineteenth-Century America," in Seizing Our Bodies: The Politics of Women's Health, ed. Claudia Dreifus (New York: Vintage Books, 1977), pp. 13-41.

34. Corea, Hidden Malpractice, pp. 268-70; Deborah Larned, "The Epidemic in Unnecessary Hysterectomy," in Seizing Our Bodies: The Politics of Women's Health, ed. Claudia Dreifus (New York: Vintage Books, 1977), pp. 195-208; McCleery et al., One Life-One Physician, pp. 8-20; and Barbara Seaman and Gideon Seaman, Women and the Crisis in Sex Hormones (New York: Bantam, 1977), pp. 373-74.

35. Margaret A. Campbell, Why Would a Girl Go into Medicine? (Old Westbury, N.Y.: Feminist Press, 1973), pp. 23, 25, 38.

36. Patricia G. Bourne and Norma J. Wikler, "Commitment and the Cultural Mandate: Women in Medicine," Social Problems 25 (April 1978): 430-40.

37. Josephine J. Williams, "Patients and Prejudice: Lay Attitudes toward Women Physicians," American Journal of Sociology 51 (January 1946): 283-87.

38. Campbell, Why Would a Girl Go into Medicine?, pp. 22-44; and Corea, Hidden Malpractice, pp. 42-44.

39. Janet M. Cuca, "The Specialization and Career Preferences of Women and Men Recently Graduated from U.S. Medical Schools," Journal of the American Medical Women's Association 34 (November 1979): 430.

40. Kathryn M. Lane, "Sex Differences in the Effect of a Surgery Clerkship on Specialty Choice," Paper presented at American Association of Medical Colleges' annual meetings, November 1979.

41. Campbell, Why Would a Girl Go into Medicine?, p. 28.

42. Statistical Abstract of the United States, 99th edition (Washington, D.C.: U.S. Bureau of the Census, 1978), p. 104.

43. See, for example, Campbell, Why Would a Girl Go into Medicine?, pp. 71-75; Corea, Hidden Malpractice, pp. 85-284.

44. Jacqueline Wallen, Howard Waitzkin, and John D. Stoeckle, "Physician Stereotypes about Female Health and Illness: A Study of Patient's Sex and the Informative Process during Medical Interviews," Women and Health 4 (Summer 1979): 135-46.

45. Diane Scully and Pauline Bart, "A Funny Thing Happened on the Way to the Orifice: Women in Gynecology Textbooks," American Journal of Sociology 78 (1973): 1045-50; and Kay Weiss, "What Medical Students Learn about Women," in Seizing Our Bodies: The Politics of Women's Health, ed. Claudia Dreifus (New York: Vintage, 1977), pp. 212-22.

46. Lewis, Fein, and Mechanic, A Right to Health, pp. 3-32.

47. Linda H. Aiken, Charles E. Lewis, John Craig, Robert C. Mendenhall, Robert J. Blendon, and David E. Rogers, "The Contribution of Specialists to the Delivery of Primary Care," New England Journal of Medicine 300 (June 1979): 1363-70.

48. Joseph A. Califano, Jr., "The Government-Medical Education Partnership," Journal of Medical Education 54 (January 1979): 19-24.

49. Ibid.

50. David Kotelchuck, "The Health Status of Americans," in Prognosis Negative: Crisis in the Health Care System, ed. David Kotelchuck (New York: Vintage, 1976), pp. 6-16.

2

PREVIOUS RESEARCH
AND PRESENT PREDICTIONS

Previous research provides a foundation for conceptualizing
most studies, even if only as a point of departure. The study reported
here is no exception; many of the ideas generated are reactions to
and elaborations of other studies of medical students. Therefore,
previous research on medical students is reviewed in this chapter in
order to give some of the theoretical underpinnings for the present
study and to demonstrate support for the hypotheses generated by the
author.

As stated previously, this study has two timely goals: (1) to
describe the effect that medical education has on medical students'
values and expectations pertaining to four health-care problem areas,
and (2) to suggest the possible implications for health care, medical
education, and the medical profession of the recent increase in the
proportion of women in medicine. The impact that women will have
on medicine is dependent in part on whether they will differ in their
professional orientations from their male colleagues. Expected orientation differences between the male and female medical students in
this study are formulated after presenting evidence of sex differences
among physicians historically and among medical students and doctors in previous research. Personality, political outlook, and other
differences between the sexes are offered as possible explanations
for the variations between males' and females' professional values.
The author proposes that initial sex differences will persist and perhaps widen through training since evidence indicates that the socialization experience of women and men may not be the same.

In order to evaluate the effect of medical education on attitudinal
change, previous research concerning professional socialization in
medical school is reviewed. Different theories concerning the fate
of values in medical school are elaborated with their varying explana-

tions for why changes may or may not result from this intense period of acculturation. With supporting evidence from previous research, the author will suggest specific values that are expected among medical students initially, expected changes in values over time, and explanations for why value changes are likely to occur. Beginning with a description of medical students upon entrance to school, the author describes students' expected views concerning problems in the doctor/patient relationship, the political and economic organization of the profession, the treatment of women, and the distribution of physicians.

INITIAL ORIENTATIONS

Since previous studies of medical students have examined only some of the specific values focused on in this study, predictions will be somewhat limited concerning the values expected among freshman medical students in North Carolina. Although medical schools have been criticized for their lack of attention to the social and psychological aspects of patient care, most medical students begin their training recognizing the importance of these factors in medical treatment.[1] Because it is in vogue to give at least lip service to dealing with the human side of patient care, most students are expected to consider rapport with patients and social and psychological factors as necessary for good medicine. However, this does not necessarily mean that in practice they will follow through on these patient-care ideals.

Studies also indicate that most medical students enter school extremely idealistic, expressing a desire to help people.[2] Although students in the present study are also expected to hold idealistic goals, when confronted with a commitment to helping people through political and social change and to working in free clinics and underserved areas, a less enthusiastic response is expected. Medical students may have a vague desire to help people on an individual basis, but they may not express interest in changing the medical system or making personal sacrifices for public good. By delineating the practical and social limitations of idealism, the author questions the assumption that professionals are altruistic and committed to social service.

Along with being idealistic, freshman medical students have traditionally expressed little interest in income and status.[3] Because it is socially taboo to openly show concern for money and prestige, students in the present study are expected to also deny interest in these pecuniary achievements. Although most students may deny personal monetary and status motivations, far fewer are expected to favor the lowering of physicians' high incomes and status. Contrasting students' personal economic motivations for entering medicine with their attitudes toward the amount of money and prestige deserved by physicians is expected to reveal a more realistic picture of entering medical students than has previous research.

In a recent study, first-year medical students were found to be about equally divided on the issue of using taxes to pay for health-care services,[4] as compared with freshman medical students and physicians in the past, who have been somewhat more opposed to any system of socialized medicine or government intervention in health care.[5] Another recent study of medical students has shown that most of the students are liberal on issues concerning government involvement in reforming (although not radically changing) the organization of medical care.[6] Students in the present study are generally expected to be about equally divided on issues of government intervention in health care, like medical students in the more recent studies, owing to the rise in political consciousness in the last decade. Students are further expected to espouse liberal values more than personal plans to work for change.

Older studies of medical students indicate that specialization is a long term trend.[7] Recent research, however, suggests that primary-care careers are experiencing an upsurge in popularity among medical students due to a greater interest in health-care delivery.[8] This trend holds for freshman medical students as well so that among entering medical students nationally in 1975, 49 percent chose primary-care fields.[9] Past studies have shown a strong correlation between rural background and choosing primary-care medicine.[10] Because many students in the present study are from rural areas and two of the three medical schools studied emphasize primary care in their selection processes, medical students in North Carolina are expected to show a strong interest in primary-care practice upon entrance to school.

Along with a growing interest in primary-care medicine, recently there seems to be a greater commitment to rural and small-town practices among medical students.[11] Because students with rural backgrounds seem more interested in practicing in rural areas than those from more urban settings,[12] medical students in North Carolina are expected to start school somewhat interested in rural practices. Inner-city ghetto practice is not expected to be a popular choice among these medical students.

Since previous research on medical students has neglected issues concerning the treatment of women physicians and patients and the need for more egalitarian doctor/patient relationships, it is difficult to predict medical students' initial values on these health-care problems. One might expect medical students to have some awareness of instances of discrimination toward women because of the women's movement, although many may not have had exposure to the specific examples focused on here. Although physicians have been criticized for their excessive authority when dealing with patients, it is unclear if entering medical students have even thought about the issue of doctor/patient equality. Thus, when first beginning this study, the author pictured freshman medical students as somewhat liberal on political and economic issues and extremely idealistic (and perhaps naive) in their plans to help others, to pay attention to social and psychological aspects of health care, and to practice primary-care and rural medicine.

PROFESSIONAL SOCIALIZATION

The process of professional socialization, including the values and perspectives that are transmitted during medical education, has been described in numerous studies of medical students.[13] Two predominately different descriptions have emerged; one indicates that during medical school students acquire values appropriate to becoming physicians, and the other proposes that many values held by students do not change and those that do may be in response to the medical school environment and not to the field of medicine. Therefore some authors describe professional socialization as an orderly process of value acquisition where students start with diverging views about medicine and the physician's role and end up with more homogeneous opinions;[14] others envision a more problematic process.[15] Likewise, the first view of socialization conceives of students as junior colleagues adopting the values of their mentors whereas the second view emphasizes the inherent conflict between students and faculty.

In a longitudinal study of medical students, Eron contends that increased cynicism and decreased humanitarianism from freshman to senior year are indicative of profound changes resulting from medical education.[16] Professional socialization is seen as a homogenizing process because students are more alike during their senior year than during their freshman year. Furthermore, other studies suggest that seniors are less interested in helping others and in dealing with patients' social and emotional problems than students in other years of training.[17]

On the other hand, Becker and his colleagues—the main proponents of the problematic view of socialization—explain changes in students' values during medical school as adjustments to the student role and not as permanent value shifts.[18] Therefore, although students may become cynical about the daily details of getting through training, it is argued that they do not lose their long-term idealistic perspective, that is, their desire to help people and their positive image of medicine. In support of this contention, one study has found that cynicism decreased for all physicians when they went into practice, especially among those whose practices involved a lot of patient contact.[19] Thus, cynicism is considered situational in nature—useful in medical school but not in medical practice.

It is difficult to come to any composite description of the socialization process based on these medical student studies. As noted previously, the way such concepts as idealism and cynicism are measured varies greatly from one study to the next. These concepts range from measuring one's perception of human nature to one's view of medical practice. Thus, it is difficult to compare the findings from studies using the same concepts measured in different ways. Also, because many of these studies measure vague values that elicit socially approved responses, we are left wondering about the effect that medical education has on values with greater relevance for patient care.

It is certainly conceivable that the homogenizing and problematic descriptions of professional socialization are both somewhat accurate, depending upon the specific values that are studied, the way that values are measured, and the particular medical school that is sampled. For example, students may maintain their idealistic desire to help people through training but may become more realistic about the ways they plan to accomplish this goal. It is certainly possible that students will come closer to adopting traditional professional views on some issues but not on others. Medical students are not likely to react like sponges, accepting all popular ideologies, but at the same time they are probably not impervious to influence from their colleagues and mentors. Examining specific professional values and expectations should help pinpoint the kinds of issues on which students have been most and least influenced during medical school.

Attitudinal change may result from most people changing their views in a uniform direction, individuals fluctuating in their opinions so that they change in opposite directions, or some combination of the two. The effects of professional socialization are most obvious on issues where students change uniformly over time. Although ignored in previous research, the different types of changes that occur on professional orientations from freshman to senior year in medical school will be specified in this study. It is hoped that describing changes in specific health-care-related orientations will provide a more realistic depiction of the socialization process than have previous studies, shed new light on the problematic versus homogenizing views of professional socialization, and suggest ways this process may eventually affect patient care.

Students have not been studied past their senior year; as a result it will not be possible to determine if attitudinal changes occur in response to medical school and therefore do not reflect lasting changes. It seems likely that even more pervasive attitudinal shifts occur when students enter practice. They may not be able to live up to their patient-care ideals when confronted with the difficulties of medical practice. Time pressures may preclude the type of doctor/patient relationship that many viewed as preferable while in medical school. Unfortunately, these issues reach beyond the scope of this study.

Medical schools have been described as conservative institutions that either ignore or exacerbate such problems as poor doctor/patient communication, geographic and specialty maldistribution of physicians, and rising medical costs.[20] If so, it seems reasonable that medical training will tend to have a conservative effect on students and will tend to make them less committed to practices based on patient needs. The specific changes that are expected from first to last year on professional values and expectations are enumerated below with explanations for why these changes may occur.

On values related to the doctor/patient relationship most studies indicate that medical students become at least somewhat less benevolent and more cynical as they go through training , whether or not these changes are considered situational adjustments to medical school school.[21] Although students become somewhat less idealistic, the majority still express interest in helping people during their senior year. Medical students in the present study are also expected to place somewhat less importance on helping people from their freshman to senior year; however, the majority of students are still expected to show interest in these socially approved ideals despite this general decline.

If seniors become more realistic in appraising their colleagues' and their own limitations, they may view criticisms of physicians' judgments more favorably than they did as freshmen. One study does indicate that seniors are more honest in realizing their own abilities and limitations than freshmen.[22] Criticisms of physicians may not seem so taboo once students actually see the mistakes physicians make and realize the shortcomings of professional knowledge.

Physicians have been criticized for perpetuating the ideology of "doctor knows best" while ignoring ways to facilitate patient understanding of medical problems. Since medical education does not emphasize doctor/patient communication, over time students may place less importance on giving information to patients concerning diagnosis and treatment as they get caught up in learning the more technical aspects of medicine. There has been no research, however, to either support or negate this contention.

Medical schools have been criticized for teaching students how to treat diseases rather than patients. Little time in the medical curriculum is spent on how to establish rapport with patients or how to deal with the psychological and social dynamics of illness. Research results are inconsistent concerning how students change on the importance they attach to humanizing doctor/patient contacts. Whereas some findings suggest that seniors place less importance on the social and psychological aspects of patient care, [23] others indicate no decreased concern with having the ability to establish rapport with patients or to get involved with patients' personal problems. [24] Because it is socially desirable to express interest in comprehensive health care, students in North Carolina are expected to profess interest in humanizing doctor/patient interactions throughout their medical training. Students have few role models for comprehensive health care; their ideals concerning the need to establish rapport with patients and to pay attention to patients' social and psychological problems may not be realized once they begin medical practice.

Students are expected to become more conservative on values related to political and economic change in medicine due in part to the conservative nature of the medical profession. Medicine represents a powerful interest group whose claims for autonomy and large financial rewards are best served by maintaining the status quo. The closer students get to joining the ranks of the medical profession, the more their interests become synonomous with supporting the existing power structure. As one arm of the medical profession, it seems likely that medical schools will perpetuate conservative ideologies in their training of medical students.

Government intervention in health care and any system of socialized medicine have long been opposed by the medical profession, since these changes might limit both the profession's control over health care and its claims for status and large financial rewards. One recent study shows that after four years of training medical students become somewhat more conservative on a wide variety of issues concerning the practice of medicine, including the question of using taxes to pay for health care. [25] Seniors in North Carolina are expected to be less in favor of government intervention in health care, changing the profit organization of the health-care system, reducing the income and prestige of doctors, working for political and social change in medicine, and doing volunteer work than they were as freshmen. The closer students get to becoming members of the medical profession, the more these liberal issues and activities conflict with their personal and professional interests. Students are expected to decline only slightly, on vague goals of humanitarian service; however, on specific plans to help people through volunteer and political work, students' interests are expected to wane more dramatically.

Along with students becoming somewhat less idealistic and more conservative through training, income and status may take on greater importance as students get closer to medical practice. One study shows that seniors are slightly more concerned than freshmen with their future income.[26] Medical students in the present study are also expected to express greater interest in money and status over time. It is anticipated that despite this expected increase in financial concerns, relatively few seniors will admit to holding these socially undesirable values. Students' interests in finances are probably better gauged by their reluctance to decrease the amount of money and status earned by physicians. Money and status may not be important reasons for choosing and staying in medicine, but upon completion of medical school few students are expected to favor lowering physicians' large financial and status rewards.

The author knows of no studies that show medical students' awareness of discrimination against women physicians and patients, because these issues have only recently come to public attention. Although a conservative trend is predicted on questions of political and economic change in medicine, the author expects that over time students will become more aware of the problems facing women physicians and patients. Now that there are more women in medical school, women's issues may have greater saliency than ever before. The presence of women's organizations, women's support groups, and vocal women who are willing to complain about sexism in the classroom may sensitize all students to the problems women face in a male-dominated profession. One study asking medical students their views toward increasing the number of black medical students shows that seniors are more in favor of an increase than freshmen.[27] This trend toward increased sympathy for minority representation is expected on women's issues as well.

As mentioned previously, recent research suggests that primary-care medicine is experiencing an upsurge in popularity among medical students. Even though more students have chosen primary-care practices in the last decade, most studies also indicate that there is a tendency toward specialization as students progress through medical training.[28] Since students are taught for the most part by specialists, they are clearly lacking in primary-care role models. Students are subjected to the biases of those who have chosen to specialize (such as, blaming incompetent medical care on primary-care physicians and learning primarily about rare diseases seen mostly in specialty practice). Students get the message that primary-care doctors, particularly those in family medicine, are less competent and less prestigious than those in specialty practice and that primary care is less interesting than specialty medicine. In fact, one study shows that medical students rank general practice lowest of all specialties in terms of status.[29] In addition to lower status, primary-care physicians generally make less money and work longer hours than specialists. Therefore, it will not be surprising if medical students in the present study tend to lose some of their initial interest in primary-care medicine.

Although admission committees at many medical schools have tried to choose students interested in rural medicine, the issue of geographic maldistribution is generally ignored once students begin their training. Because so much of medical training today is dependent on complex medical technology, students are not prepared for practices in rural areas where little technology is available. Students probably choose practice locations based less on the needs of patients than on personal needs, the desirability of the patient population in terms of education and income, and the wish for professional colleagues, decent working hours, medical equipment, and hospital facilities. Many factors appear to mitigate against the selection of a location based solely on patient need. One study of medical students shows that freshmen are more interested in rural practice than seniors,[30] although another study finds no relationship between year in school and interest in rural medicine.[31] The author expects that medical students in North Carolina will become increasingly less committed to practices based on patient need and will therefore become less interested in rural and inner-city medicine from freshman to senior year.

Some reasons have been described for the predicted conservative trends and loss of interest in patient need among medical students as a whole. These reasons stem from the conservative and non-public health orientation of medical education and the medical profession. Based on previous research and on interviews conducted with a select number of medical students, the author has specified some factors related to experiences in medical school that may explain why particular students' values change over time. It is proposed that conservative and nonhumanitarian professional orientation changes might be due to low grades, substantial school debts, being treated badly by faculty, experiencing difficulty in school, accepting how physicians treat patients, lack of familiarity with or opposition to the women's movement, not participating in liberal organizations, becoming more conservative in political outlook, lacking ideological support from peers, expecting to do academic medicine or specialty practice, perceiving discouragement for primary-care medicine, tending to agree with faculty on political issues in medicine, and viewing one's career negatively. Some other background factors tested to see if they might also explain changes in orientation over time are students' medical school, marital status, parental status (whether they are parents or not), age, father's education, urban/rural background, religion, race, and sex. The results of the data analysis indicating whether any of these explanatory variables accounts for changes in medical students' professional orientations are presented in Chapter 6. Although numerous other factors may also account for attitudinal change, these have been omitted, since some were too difficult or impossible to measure (such as maturing), some were not related to the experience of medical school (and thus considered less important in a study of professional socialization), and some were relevant to medical education but limitations in questionnaire length did not allow for their inclusion.

Thus far, previous research concerning the professional orientation of freshman medical students and changes in these orientations from first to last year in medical school has been reviewed. Hypotheses stemming from previous research have also been enumerated, indicating what changes in professional orientation are expected and why these fluctuations may occur.

Besides interest in the values and expectations that medical students as a whole bring to their training, the author is also concerned with how and why male and female students might differ on these orientations initially and how professional socialization might affect the sexes differently. Therefore, in the next section of this chapter a brief history of women in medicine and previous studies comparing males and females in medicine are presented as support for sex differences expected on professional orientations initially and over time.

COMPARISONS OF MEN AND WOMEN

There were two main groups of women doctors in the early part of this century: a small militant group concerned with equal opportunity for women doctors, improvement in health care for women patients, and social change in medicine; and a larger more conservative group that identified with upper-class professional interests more than with women. [32] Like the women's movement historically, class loyalties prevented most women in medicine from uniting with women patients on common concerns.

Whether feminist or not, women physicians have done research on many women's diseases and problems ignored by male physicians. For example, the first woman doctor in Holland helped develop the diaphragm because she was concerned that women were suffering from too many pregnancies. This research occurred at a time when many doctors were afraid that birth control would decrease the number of available patients. Another woman doctor, Dorothy Mendenhall, became interested in research on ways to reduce infant mortality after her own child died from bad but accepted obstetrical practice. [33] It seems that women doctors in the past have been more oriented than male physicians to health problems affecting women and that today they may show more concern with protecting women from such malpractices as medical experimentation and unnecessary surgery.

Although difficult to prove, it seems likely that research priorities can be affected by the personal and monetary interests of those who design and fund the research. This is most obvious in the case of the Dalkon Shield, a birth control device later proved extremely unsafe for women. Because women suffered from the faulty Dalkon Shield and not male drug company executives or researchers, we might expect a less cautious attitude than if the birth control device had been meant for male consumption. In fact, it was a woman doctor who first suggested to the researchers that the Dalkon Shield was unsafe. (One wonders whether it would have taken many deaths and hundreds of painful operations before the device was taken off the market if it had been originally designed for men or had it not made so much money for the researchers who created it.) One argument for minority representation in medicine is to help protect minorities from experimentation and the abuses that the profit motive encourages.[34]

In addition to showing concern for women's health problems, women physicians have also demonstrated some interest in public health and social change in medicine. Although few physicians choose public health medicine, women physicians have been more likely to select this field than men.[35] Women doctors have been at the forefront of social change in medicine in such areas as preventive, psychosomatic, and occupational medicine. In comparing male and female medical organizations, one finds that the American Medical Association (AMA) has always taken conservative stands on issues of political and economic reform in medicine. However, the American Medical Women's Association (the female counterpart of the AMA) has a history of progressive stances on such reforms as medicare and medicaid.[36]

Because only a small proportion of women doctors have been members of the American Medical Women's Association, have chosen to work in public health or for social change, or have shown special interest in the problems of women, most women physicians have followed the mainstream of American medicine like their male colleagues. In the past, class loyalties have generally been stronger than sex loyalties so that the majority of women doctors have identified more closely with the interests of the profession than with those of working-class women. This is not to deny the progressive accomplishments of women physicians, such as those already mentioned, but to add a note of caution to the assumption that women will necessarily be responsive to public health needs. Because women have traditionally been in a precarious position in the profession and have had to fight for acceptance, trying to blend into the mainstream of medicine was probably a better survival tactic than confronting the inequalities in the system. Now that there are more women in medicine, we may find that proportionally more women doctors will be interested in the problems experienced by women and poor patients than in the past.

Finding more acceptance in medicine, women doctors may be more willing to rock the boat.

Due in part to the previous scarcity of women in the field there has been little research comparing males and females in medicine on issues relevant to health care; recently, however, more studies have focused on sex differences. Existing research on women medical students and physicians has been primarily concerned with the problems women face in a male profession and with the difficulties involved with balancing career and family commitments.[37] The studies described next compare the sexes on professional orientations similar to those focused on in the present study.

Recently there has been speculation that women will add a needed touch of humanity to medicine due to the greater nurturance and empathy associated with the traditional female role. Studies of medical students, medical school applicants, and physicians have conflicting findings with regard to the contention that women are more nurturant and idealistic than men. Some find that women score higher on nurturance,[38] whereas others indicate either that men and women are equally nurturant and interested in helping people,[39] or that women possess less of these characteristics than men.[40] Although the evidence is contradictory, the author proposes that, upon entrance to medical school, female medical students in North Carolina will show greater interest in helping people than their male counterparts.

Some evidence exists that, among medical students and physicians, women are also more interested than men in the psychological factors in illness and in establishing close patient relationships.[41] In the present study, female medical students are initially expected to place greater importance than their male peers on the social and psychological aspects of patient care, including the need to establish rapport with clients. Women are therefore expected to have a humanizing impact on the medical profession and on the practice of medicine.

Little research has dealt with values aimed at equalizing the doctor/patient relationship and at reducing professional dominance. One study of first-year Swedish medical students in 1960 shows that women are more likely than men to value giving information to patients concerning diagnosis and treatment.[42] This is consistent with previous studies indicating women's desire for close patient contacts and with a recent study suggesting that women physicians are more open and honest with dying patients and tend to communicate better than male physicians.[43] Among freshman medical students in North Carolina, women are expected to support more egalitarian doctor/patient relationships than are the men. Specifically, women are predicted to place more importance on providing health information to patients about diagnosis and treatment and to be more critical of absolute patient confidence in physicians.

Besides expecting women to show greater interest than men in humanitarian and egalitarian relationships with patients, they are also expected to more strongly advocate political and economic reform in medicine. A recent study of physicians shows that women are more liberal than men on scales of political outlook and medical politics, even after controlling for age. [44] One study of successful medical applicants also shows that women score higher than men on a personality inventory measuring change and social service. [45]

In studies of medical students, medical applicants, and physicians, women have been shown to be much less interested in high income and status than men. [46] In fact, in a recent study of physicians the author demonstrates that women receive lower fees than men for the same procedures. [47] Although this finding is interpreted as an indication of discrimination against women, it seems reasonable that lower fees from women reflect their lower concern with money, because doctors, and not patients, set pay schedules. Although some feminists may take exception with this latter interpretation, the author considers that charging lower fees is not only reasonable but beneficial for patients since physicians' charges are often too exorbitant for most to afford.

Along with being less oriented to money, women have always been more likely to take salaried work. [48] Advocating reforms like socialized medicine and reducing physicians' status and income are probably less threatening to those who are salaried and to those who are less interested in the economic rewards of medicine. Therefore, the author expects that among first-year medical students, women will be more likely than men to plan volunteer work and to advocate government intervention to both reduce professional control over health care and lower the income and status of physicians.

Another reason why women are expected to show greater interest in working for and advocating political and economic reform in medicine is because minority status often promotes liberal values. [49] It is easier to be sympathetic with those lacking power who are pushing for change if one is also part of a group experiencing discrimination. Furthermore, because medicine is an untraditional career choice for women, politically liberal women are probably self-selected into medical school. The women's movement may also have politicized women about issues other than those specifically related to women. The women's health movement has been concerned with the need for change in the political and economic organization of medicine, and not just women's rights. Women may be concerned with changing the medical profession if they realize the connection between women's medical care and the health-care system.

Upon entrance to school, female medical students are expected to be more aware than their male peers of discrimination toward women physicians and patients. Not surprisingly, one study of medical students indicates that females are more supportive than males of women's rights to work and to have careers.[50] Likewise, another study of physicians shows that women are more liberal on medical feminism than men.[51] It is in the self-interest of women medical students to be aware of discrimination against women physicians and patients. Personal experiences and contact with the literature and rhetoric of the women's movement have probably sensitized women to issues concerning their sex. For example, having been gynecological patients, females are probably more familiar than males with the tendency of physicians to treat female patients in a patronizing and insensitive way. Issues of discrimination toward women are therefore expected to be more salient for women medical students.

Finally, with regard to primary-care and location-of-practice intentions, only sex differences on location plans are expected. A study of recent medical school graduates nationally shows little difference between the sexes on plans to practice primary-care medicine.[52] When these graduates were asked about their motivations for choosing a specialty based on societal need, the same study found basically no sex difference.

In recent surveys of medical students, women were slightly less likely than men to choose a rural or small-town practice at some schools studied.[53] National data on medical school graduates in 1978 did not, however, indicate a sex difference on rural practice plans.[54] It seems plausible that women would be less interested in rural practice for several reasons. First, women may feel that locating in a rural area is more difficult because they may more often be required to consider a spouse's career when deciding where to settle. Moreover, because there is a marriage gradient in our society, that is, women tend to marry men of higher socioeconomic status and men tend to marry women of lower status,[55] being in a rural area may seem even more socially limiting for an unmarried woman than for an unmarried man. For these reasons, men might be more likely to plan a rural practice than women.

National data on medical school graduates in 1978 did show women to have slightly more interest than men in inner-city ghetto practice.[56] For some women who want to meet critical health needs, inner-city locations may seem more favorable than rural areas.

Testable Explanations of
Initial Sex Differences

Most sociological studies comparing males and females make little attempt to go beyond a simple description of differences. The fact that one sex may possess more or less of a particular quality does not tell us what it is about being a woman or a man that leads to these sex differences. Therefore, the present study will make some attempt to explain why it is that the sexes differ in their professional orientation upon entrance to medical school. Explanations to account for these sex variations will also be tested.

To begin, the author will determine if sex differences among freshmen can be explained by variations between the sexes in their social origins or backgrounds. For example, if women are more liberal on political and economic issues, it may because proportionally more of them are from upper-class families where liberal values are more commonly endorsed. In this case, women medical students' more liberal stance would be explained by their social-class backgrounds and not their sex. Thus variables pertaining to students' backgrounds and origins are held constant in order to control for other possible explanations of the findings.

Particular background characteristics were selected for control variables because previous research indicated that they might be associated with certain professional orientations or because interviews with first-year medical students suggested these factors as having influenced students' views. The following social background characteristics have been included in this study in order to determine if they account for the initial sex differences in professional orientation: race, religion, religiosity, marital status, age, rural/urban background, father's education, father's socioeconomic status, age decided to study medicine, presence and number of physicians in one's family, presence of physician father and physician friends, and the amount of debt expected upon completion of training. The initial sex differences on professional values and expectations are not expected to be caused by differences between the sexes on these social background characteristics.

If the sex differences are not explained by a dissimilarity in social background, then the author will determine whether the sex effect on professional orientation reflects more general value differences between males and females. As suggested before, traditional sex-role socialization may contribute to such sex differences as women being more nurturant, less dominant, less competitive, and less interested in money and status than are men. Personality differences between men and women attributed to early sex-role socialization are documented in most studies of medical students, medical applicants, and college students. On personality inventories, women tend to score higher on nurturance and lower on dominance and competitiveness than men.[57] Women may advocate more humanitarian and egalitarian relationships with patients as well as more liberal stances on other values due to personality traits associated with growing up female.

For example, it can be argued that women will want to restrict professional autonomy and physicians' income and status more than men because they are taught to be less dominant and less interested in money. Likewise, women's greater nurturance may explain their greater emphasis on the social and psychological factors in health care. These propositions will be tested in this research.

An implicit assumption of much medical student research is that a cynical world view affects one's professional values. Because women are expected to express more idealistic reasons for choosing medicine, they may also be less cynical in their world view than men. Cynicism is therefore included as another personality variable that may explain the sex differences on professional orientations. For example, men may be more interested in making large incomes because they tend to view life more cynically.

As stated previously, because medicine is a deviant career choice for women and a conformist choice for men, we might expect that women medical students will be more politically liberal than the men. Women are to some extent pioneers in a male profession. As shown before, one study of physicians shows that women are more politically liberal than men. Because minority status is expected to promote liberalism, the author expects that some of the initial sex differences on political, economic, and women's issues in medicine will reflect women's more liberal political outlook.

As mentioned previously, we might also expect women to be more liberal than men due to the politicizing influence of the women's movement. The women's movement has helped keep the political issues of the 1960s and 1970s alive for women whereas no comparable social movement has done this for men. Unfortunately, the author neglected to ask questions concerning involvement with the women's movement in the first questionnaire administered during the freshman year. Therefore, we can only speculate on the influence that this social movement may have had on students' orientations before entering medical school.

Another possible explanation of the sex differences is women's minority status in general and their anticipation of being a minority in a predominantly male profession. Minority status probably plays an important role in the acquisition of liberal values, since it is in the interests of less powerful groups to advocate change in the status quo. The experience of being a minority person is difficult to measure directly using survey techniques. Therefore, minority status and contact with the women's movement are posed as residual or untested explanations for the initial sex differences on professional orientations.

The following factors were thus expected to at least partially explain sex differences in professional orientations upon entrance to medical school: (1) personality traits (nurturance, dominance, cynicism, and competitiveness), (2) general political outlook, (3) the importance of high status and income, (4) anticipation of minority status in the profession and minority status in general, and (5) contact with the ideas of the women's movement. Only the first three categories above are actually tested in this research.

The Fate of Sex Differences

Because males and females differ initially in their professional orientations, the next question is, Will these differences persist over time or will professional socialization have a leveling effect on attitudinal variations? Although numerous studies have focused on the topic of professional socialization, none have systematically examined how this process may differ for males and females in medical school.

As stated before, studies portray diverging images of the socialization process; some describe an orderly process whereby students acquire dominant professional ideologies and others argue that medical school does not produce lasting attitudinal shifts. Professional socialization in medical school may be less orderly and more problematic for such minorities as women due to some of the difficulties that they face in a predominantly male profession. Therefore a description of the socialization process should take into account how this process may vary for such minorities as women.

Recently, there have been numerous publications detailing the problems that women physicians and students encounter in the medical profession. [58] Problems often mentioned center around women's exclusion from colleagueship and the sponsorship system due to the "men's club" atmosphere in most medical schools. Women medical students report numerous examples of overt and subtle discrimination by male peers and faculty, although a recent study suggests that at least overt sex discrimination is on the decline. [59] More subtle types of discrimination, such as sexist jokes, and acts of omission, like exclusion from informal learning experiences, suggest that medicine is not a place for women. More specific examples of discrimination toward women were given in Chapter 1.

Women medical students have coped with discrimination in a variety of ways. Some deny its existence or perhaps are even unaware of sexism in medicine. Many of these women may actively try to become "one of the boys" or "better men" in order to avoid notice. Of those who are aware of discrimination, some have tried to constructively deal with these problems. Women's support groups and organizations have formed in many medical schools in response to the difficulties women face in a male-dominated profession.

Whether as a reaction to discrimination or not, a previous study reports that women tend to see medical school as a job and thus try to maintain a separate identity; men tend to identify themselves with the medical student role. [60] Thus, there is evidence that women are less integrated into medical school than men.

The relative isolation of women, the scarcity of female role models, and the formation of alternative support groups suggest that socialization in the medical profession may be a less orderly process resulting in less conformity to professional values for women than for men. This may not be the case for women who try to become "one of the boys" by adopting dominant professional values. The author proposes that although some women in North Carolina medical schools may deny their common interests as minority members in the profession, most will participate in or at least be sympathetic with alternative women's reference groups advocating values that may differ from those of the male-dominated profession. There is considerable debate over the, "degree to which women who are interested in medical careers can undergo the traditional male physician-dominated professional socialization process and remain feminist in orientation."[61] This author expects that feminism may buffer the effects of professional socialization.

Thus differences between males and females on professional orientations are expected to persist or even widen over time due to women's contact with the women's movement and related literature of the women's health movement and to their participation in liberal organizations in medical school. Because the literature of the women's health movement, such as Our Bodies, Ourselves,[62] takes a politically liberal stance as well as a profeminist view, contact with these women's ideologies is expected to have a broadly politicizing and humanizing impact on those familiar with it. If women have greater contact with the women's health movement literature and with liberal and minority organizations in medicine, then we should expect them to maintain a more liberal outlook through their training as compared to men. This study will test these contentions by exploring why males and females may change differently in their professional orientations over time. Thus, the original sex differences on professional values may widen or at least persist because socialization is not expected to be a great leveler of attitudes. Because of the scarcity of studies comparing women and men through medical training, there is no empirical evidence that either supports or refutes these hypotheses.

Women may have a beneficial impact on the profession, medical education, and patient care if in the senior year they are more aware than men of problems in health-care delivery and quality and if they are more likely to advocate reforms that address these problems. Women may provide good role models for their colleagues by pointing out the importance of developing egalitarian relationships with patients, marked by good communication and rapport. Because some of the worst complaints leveled at the medical profession have concerned the doctor/patient relationship, the increase in the proportion of women in medicine may add a needed touch of humanity.

If women show more concern than men about discrimination toward women in medicine, it seems likely that their presence will contribute to improved conditions for women physicians. The treatment of women patients may also improve if in addition to being more egalitarian in treating patients, women physicians serve as nonsexist role models for other physicians.

If women more strongly advocate such reforms as socialized medicine and lower physician income, this may translate in practice to being more responsive to public health needs and to charging lower fees than men. If these predicted sex differences emerge, it seems likely that women will have a liberalizing effect on the profession of medicine, although it is not proposed that they will radically change the profession's power structure.

Because no sex differences are expected on plans to practice primary-care medicine, the recent increase of women in medicine is not expected to greatly affect specialty-maldistribution problems. If women are less interested in rural practice but more inclined toward inner-city practice, their effect on geographic maldistribution should be negligible. The recruitment of other groups underrepresented in medicine, such as blacks and those raised in rural areas, is expected to have a greater influence than sex on maldistribution problems because these groups have previously been more likely to settle in need areas.[63]

In this chapter, the author reviewed previous studies concerning professional orientations common among medical students, professional socialization during medical school, orientation differences between women and men in medical school, and differential socialization of the sexes during training. The evidence from these studies was used to generate numerous hypotheses that will be tested in this research. These pertain to students' initial orientations, changes in these orientations over four years, and sex differences on professional orientations initially and over time. By describing changes in specific health-care-related orientations and by focusing on sex differences, the author hopes to provide a more realistic depiction of medical students and the socialization process than have previous studies; shed new light on the problematic versus homogenizing views of professional socialization, particularly as this process may differ for males and females; and suggest ways that socialization and differences in professional orientation between the sexes may eventually affect medical education, the profession, and patient care. Before reporting the results of the data analysis concerning these issues, data collection and measurement information will be detailed in the following chapter.

NOTES

1. Samuel Bloom, Power and Dissent in the Medical School (New York: Free Press, 1973), pp. 75-90; Rodney M. Coe, Max Pepper, and Mary Mattis, "The 'New' Medical Student: Another View," Journal of Medical Education 52 (February 1977): 89-98; and Marcel A. Fredericks and Paul Mundy, The Making of a Physician (Chicago: Loyola University Press, 1976), pp. 37-41.

2. Howard S. Becker, Blanche Geer, Everette C. Hughes, and Anselm L. Strauss, Boys in White (Chicago: University of Chicago Press, 1961), pp. 70-79; Bloom, Power and Dissent, pp. 93-107; and Don Cahalan, Patricia Collette, and Norman A. Hilmar, "Career Interests and Expectations of U.S. Medical Students," Journal of Medical Education 32 (August 1957): 557-63.

3. Becker, et al., Boys in White, pp. 70-79; Bloom, Power and Dissent, pp. 93-107; Cahalan, Collette, and Hilmar, "Career Interests and Expectations," pp. 557-63.

4. Coe, Pepper, and Mattis, "The 'New' Medical Student," pp. 89-98.

5. John Colombotos, "Social Origins and Ideology of Physicians: A Study of the Effects of Early Socialization," Journal of Health and Social Behavior 10 (March 1969): 16-29; and Fredericks and Mundy, Making of a Physician, pp. 37-41.

6. Lee Goldman, "Factors Related to Physicians' Medical and Political Attitudes: A Documentation of Intraprofessional Variations," Journal of Health and Social Behavior 15 (September 1974): 177-87.

7. Patricia L. Kendall and Hanan C. Selvin, "Tendencies toward Specialization in Medical Training," in The Student-Physician: Introductory Studies in the Sociology of Medical Education, ed. Robert K. Merton, George G. Reader, and Patricia L. Kendall (Cambridge, Mass.: Harvard University Press, 1957), pp. 153-74; and Milton Terris and Mary Monk, "Changes in Physicians' Careers," Journal of the American Medical Association 160 (February 1956): 653-55.

8. Janet M. Cuca, "The Specialization and Career Preferences of Women and Men Recently Graduated from U.S. Medical Schools," Journal of the American Medical Women's Association 34 (November 1979) : 425-35; and Daniel H. Funkenstein, Medical Students, Medical Schools and Society during Five Eras: Factors Affecting the Career Choices of Physicians 1958-1976 (Cambridge, Mass.: Ballinger, 1978), pp. 5-71.

9. The percentage choosing primary-care fields includes those selecting family practice, internal medicine, and pediatrics among

1975 freshmen who had decided on a field. The percentages were calculated so that the undecided freshmen and those with no opinion were excluded from the total. See W. F. Dubé, Descriptive Study of Enrolled Medical Students 1975-6 (Washington, D. C.: Association of American Medical Colleges, 1977), pp. 67-68.

10. See, for example, Richard Oates and Harry Feldman, "Patterns of Change in Medical Student Career Choices," Journal of Medical Education 49 (1974): 562-69.

11. Funkenstein, Medical Students, Medical Schools and Society, pp. 88-98; and Marie R. Haug, Bebe Lavin, and Naomi Breslau, "Practice Location Preferences at Entry to Medical School," Journal of Medical Education 55 (April 1980): 333-38.

12. Mark Taylor, William Dickman, and Robert Kane, "Medical Students' Attitudes toward Rural Practice," Journal of Medical Education 48 (October 1973): 885-95.

13. For a good review of the literature concerning professional socialization in medical school, see Agnes Rezler, "Attitude Changes during Medical School: A Review of the Literature," Journal of Medical Education 49 (November 1974): 1023-30.

14. Leonard Eron, "The Effect of Medical Education on Attitudes: A Follow-up Study," Journal of Medical Education 33, pt. 2 (October 1958): 25-33; and Robert K. Merton, George G. Reader, and Patricia L. Kendall, eds., The Student-Physician: Introductory Studies in the Sociology of Medical Education (Cambridge, Mass.: Harvard University Press, 1957).

15. Becker, et al., Boys in White, especially pp. 419-33; Isabel R. Juan, Rosalia E. A. Paiva, Harold B. Haley, and Robert O'Keefe, "High and Low Levels of Dogmatism in Relation to Personality Characteristics of Medical Students: A Follow-up Study," Psychological Reports 34 (1974): 303-15.

16. Eron, "Effect of Medical Education on Attitudes," pp. 25-33.

17. Richard Christie and Robert K. Merton, "Procedures for the Sociological Study of the Values Climate of Medical Schools," Journal of Medical Education 33, pt. 2 (October 1958): 125-53; and Leonard V. Gordon and Ivan N. Mensh, "Values of Medical School Students at Different Levels of Training," Journal of Educational Psychology 53 (1962): 48-51.

18. Becker et al., Boys in White, especially pp. 419-33.

19. Robert M. Gray, W. R. Elton Newman, and Adina M. Reinhardt, "The Effect of Medical Specialization on Physicians' Attitudes," Journal of Health and Human Behavior 7 (Summer 1966): 128-32.

20. Steven Jonas, Medical Mystery: The Training of Doctors in the United States (New York: W. W. Norton, 1978).

21. Eron, "Effect of Medical Education on Attitudes," pp. 25-33; Gordon and Mensh, "Values of Medical School Students", pp. 48-51; Juan, et al., "High and Low Levels of Dogmatism", pp. 303-15; and Pearl P. Rosenberg, "Catch 22—The Medical Model," in Becoming a Physician, ed. Eileen C. Shapiro and Leah M. Lowenstein (Cambridge, Mass.: Ballinger, 1979), pp. 81-91.

22. Edwin Rosinski, "Professional, Ethical, and Intellectual Attitudes of Medical Students," Journal of Medical Education 38 (December 1963): 1016-22.

23. Bloom, Power and Dissent, pp. 75-90; and Christie and Merton, "Procedures for the Sociological Study of Values," pp. 125-53.

24. Bloom, Power and Dissent, pp. 75-90; and Coe, Pepper, and Mattis, "The 'New' Medical Student," pp. 89-98.

25. Coe, Pepper, and Mattis, "The 'New' Medical Student," pp. 89-98.

26. Bloom, Power and Dissent, pp. 93-107.

27. Coe, Pepper, and Mattis, "The 'New' Medical Student," pp. 89-98.

28. Mark S. Plovnick, "Primary Care Career Choices and Medical Student Learning Styles," Journal of Medical Education 50 (September 1975): 849-55; and Taylor, Dickman, and Kane, "Medical Students' Attitudes," pp. 885-95.

29. Daniel B. Fishman and Carl N. Zimet, "Specialty Choice and Beliefs about Specialties among Freshman Medical Students," Journal of Medical Education 47 (July 1972): 524-33.

30. Oates and Feldman, "Patterns of Change in Medical Student Career Choices," pp. 562-69.

31. Taylor, Dickman, and Kane, "Medical Students' Attitudes," pp. 885-95.

32. Gena Corea, The Hidden Malpractice: How American Medicine Mistreats Women (New York: Jove, 1977), pp. 51-63; and Carol Lopate, Women in Medicine (Baltimore, Md.: Johns Hopkins Press, 1968), pp. 16-24.

33. Corea, Hidden Malpractice, pp. 135-55 and 210-14.

34. See Mark Dowie and Tracy Johnston, "A Case of Corporate Malpractice and the Dalkon Shield," in Seizing Our Bodies, ed. Claudia Dreifus (New York: Vintage Books, 1978), pp. 86-104.

35. Maryland V. Pennell and Josephine E. Renshaw, "Distribution of Women Physicians, 1971," Journal of the American Medical Women's Association 28 (April 1973): 181-86.

36. Lopate, Women in Medicine, pp. 16-24.

37. See, for example, Patricia G. Bourne and Norma J. Wikler, "Commitment and the Cultural Mandate: Women in Medicine,"

Social Problems 25 (April 1978): 430-40; and Margaret A. Campbell, Why Would a Girl Go into Medicine? (Old Westbury, N.Y.: Feminist Press, 1973).

38. Mary Fruen, Arthur Rothman, and Jan Steiner, "Comparison of Characteristics of Male and Female Medical School Applicants," Journal of Medical Education 49 (February 1974): 137-45; and Robert Roessler, Forrest Collins, and Roy B. Mefferd, "Sex Similarities in Successful Medical School Applicants," Journal of the American Medical Women's Association 30 (June 1975): 254-65.

39. Marshall Becker, Marilyn Katatsky, and Henry Seidel, "A Follow-up Study of Unsuccessful Applicants to Medical Schools," Journal of Medical Education 48 (November 1973): 991-1001; and Nancy G. Kutner and Donna R. Brogan, "The Decision to Enter Medicine: Motivations, Social Support, and Discouragements for Women," Psychology of Women Quarterly 5 (Winter 1980): 341-58.

40. Ellen McGrath and Carl N. Zimet, "Female and Male Medical Students: Differences in Specialty Choice Selection and Personality," Journal of Medical Education 52 (April 1977): 293-300.

41. Funkenstein, Medical Students, Medical Schools and Society, pp. 73-82; John Kosa and Robert E. Coker, Jr., "The Female Physician in Public Health: Conflict and Reconciliation of the Sex and Professional Roles," in Professional Woman, ed. Athena Theodore (Cambridge, Mass.: Schenkman, 1971), pp. 195-206; H. J. Walton, "Sex Differences in Ability and Outlook of Senior Medical Students," British Journal of Medical Education 2 (June 1968): 156-62; and H. J. Walton, J. Drewery, and G. M. Carstairs, "Interest of Graduating Medical Students in Social and Emotional Aspects of Illness," British Medical Journal, September 1963, pp. 588-92.

42. Joachim Israel and Per Sjöstrand, "Generalized Role as a Factor Influencing the Learning of Professional Values and Attitudes," Acta Sociologica 11 (1968): 177-93.

43. George E. Dickinson and Algene A. Pearson, "Sex Differences of Physicians in Relating to Dying Patients," Journal of the American Medical Women's Association 34 (January 1979): 45-47.

44. Marilyn Heins, "Career and Life Patterns of Women and Men Physicians," in Becoming a Physician, ed. Eileen C. Shapiro and Leah M. Lowenstein (Cambridge, Mass.: Ballinger, 1979), pp. 217-35.

45. Roessler, Collins, and Mefferd, "Sex Similarities," pp. 254-65.

46. Becker, Katatsky, and Seidel, "A Follow-up Study", pp. 991-1001; Cuca, "Specialization and Career Preferences," pp. 425-35; Funkenstein, Medical Students, Medical Schools and Society, pp. 73-82; Kosa and Coker, "Female Physician in Public Health," pp. 195-206; and Kutner and Brogan, "Decision to Enter Medicine," pp. 341-58.

47. Jean W. Adams, "Patient Discrimination against Women Physicians," Journal of the American Medical Women's Association 32 (July 1977): 225-61.

48. Cuca, "Specialization and Career Preferences," pp. 425-35; and Roscoe Dykman and John Stalnaker, "Survey of Women Physicians Graduating from Medical School 1925-1940," Journal of Medical Education 32 (March 1957): 3-38.

49. David Sears, "Political Behavior," in The Handbook of Social Psychology, ed. Gardner Lindzey and Elliot Aronson, vol. 5 (Reading, Mass.: Addison-Wesley, 1969), pp. 399-458.

50. R. A. Hudson Rosen, "Occupational Role Innovators and Sex Role Attitudes," Journal of Medical Education 49 (June 1974): 554-61.

51. Heins, "Career and Life Patterns," pp. 217-35.

52. Cuca, "Specialization and Career Preferences," pp. 425-35.

53. Nancy G. Kutner and Donna R. Brogan, "A Comparison of the Practice Orientations of Women and Men Students at Two Medical Schools," Journal of the American Medical Women's Association 35 (March 1980): 80-86; Haug, Lavin, and Breslau, "Practice Location Preferences at Entry to Medical School," pp. 333-38.

54. Janet M. Cuca, "1978 U.S. Medical School Graduates: Practice Setting Preferences, Other Career Plans and Personal Characteristics," Journal of Medical Education 55 (May 1980): 465-68.

55. Jessie Bernard, The Future of Marriage (New York: Bantam, 1972), pp. 35-37.

56. Cuca, "1978 U.S. Medical School Graduates," pp. 465-68.

57. Fruen, Rothman, and Steiner, "Comparison of Characteristics," pp. 137-45; Edwin B. Hutchins, Judith Reitman, and Dorothy Klaub, "Minorities, Manpower, and Medicine," Journal of Medical Education 42 (September 1967): 809-21; and Roessler, Collins, and Mefferd, "Sex Similarities," pp. 254-65.

58. See note 37 for some examples.

59. Carolyn Spieler, ed., Women in Medicine 1976 (New York: Josiah Macy, Jr., Foundation, 1977).

60. Rosenberg, "Catch 22," pp. 81-91.

61. Eileen C. Shapiro and Amber B. Jones, "Women Physicians and the Exercise of Power and Authority in Health Care," in Becoming a Physician, ed. Eileen C. Shapiro and Leah M. Lowenstein (Cambridge, Mass.: Ballinger, 1979), p. 242.

62. Boston Women's Health Book Collective, Our Bodies, Ourselves: A Book by and for Women (New York: Simon and Schuster, 1976).

63. Cuca, "1978 U.S. Medical School Graduates," pp. 465-68; Lawrence Schwartz and James R. Cantwell," Weiskotten Survey, Class of 1960: A Profile on Physician Location and Specialty Choice," Journal of Medical Education 51 (July 1976): 533-40; and Taylor, Dickman, and Kane, "Medical Students' Attitudes," pp. 885-95.

3

DATA COLLECTION
AND MEASUREMENT

This chapter presents the data collection techniques and a description of how important variables have been measured. Two questionnaires, one given to medical students during their freshman year of medical school and the other administered during the students' senior year, provided the majority of data analyzed in this longitudinal study. The two questionnaires were the culmination of numerous pretests and interviews with medical students. Because the author has devised a new conceptualization of professional values, these pretests and interviews aided in developing reliable measures of professional orientation. Interviews with medical students also pointed to experiences in medical school that might explain changes in orientation over time.

Details on the measurement of professional orientations and explanatory variables are elaborated on after the description of data collection procedures is outlined below in the research history. The measurement discussion is rather lengthy since many of the professional orientations and explanatory variables have not been previously validated. The explanatory variables include social background attributes, personality characteristics, political outlook, and measures concerning experiences in medical school. These variables have been included in the data analysis in order to account for gender differences in professional orientation upon entrance to medical school and students changes in professional orientation from freshman to senior year.

RESEARCH HISTORY

Pretests and Interviews

Since most previous research conceptions of professional values lacked specificity and relevance to health care, the author was posed

with the problem of writing a large set of reliable and valid questions
to measure each of the professional orientations outlined in Chapter 1.
After extensive reading of the studies on medical students and the critiques of the medical profession, an initial questionnaire was constructed. This questionnaire was pretested in 1974 on all first-year medical students at Duke University School of Medicine, the University of
North Carolina School of Medicine, and Bowman Gray School of Medicine. Sixty-seven percent of all students at these three schools returned the instrument.

Analysis of the interrelationships among the questions pertaining to students' professional orientations showed few obvious clusters
of items and low inter-item correlations. Higher correlations among
items of similar content were needed in order to group questions into
indexes, which tend to be more reliable than single-item measures.
A review of the questionnaire and subsequent interviews with medical
students suggested four plausible explanations for the low inter-item
correlations: the diffuse attitudinal structure of the data reflected
the uncrystalized attitudes of students upon entrance to medical school;
the lack of a neutral opinion category forced opinions where none may
have existed; the low inter-item correlations were due to ambiguously
worded questions; and too few items tapping a wide variety of issues
were included in the questionnaire, rather than many questions focusing on a select number of values. These insights from the initial
pretest aided in developing the final questionnaire that included a
neutral opinion category on many items, more clearly worded questions, and more items concerning fewer topics.

To further revise the questionnaire, it was necessary to determine which health-care issues were salient to entering medical students so that the research would reflect students' concerns as well
as those of the author. It also was important to ascertain from students' perspectives those factors contributing to their initial professional orientations so that these variables could be statistically con-
trolled in analyzing sex differences. Therefore, interviews with 13
selected medical students from Duke University were conducted in
1975 at the end of their first year in order to aid the revision of the
questionnaire and the interpretation of findings. Only Duke University
medical students were chosen since they were more accessible in
terms of proximity to the researcher and cooperation from the medical school than students at other institutions. Students who scored
high or low on designated values and expectations on the pretest were
chosen for the interview to ensure the representation of students with
a wide range of professional orientations.

As expected, the interviews aided in the revision of the questionnaire by determining which aspects of the health-care system students found problematic. Students mentioned many of the previously

reported problems with the quality and delivery of health care. For example, many complained about the elitist and God-like attitudes of physicians, geographic maldistribution of doctors, and physicians' desires for status and large incomes. These issues as well as others were included in the revised questionnaire. Some other questions on health-care problems were dropped from the questionnaire, since students either did not understand these issues or held no clear opinions on them. For instance, items concerning the delegation of authority to physician assistants and nurse midwives were omitted because students generally had little knowledge about the training of such paraprofessionals. The interviews were also a guide to understanding and measuring complex professional orientations, such as students' reluctance to admit personal status and financial motivations. Thus, items concerning how much income and prestige physicians deserve, in general, were also included in the revised questionnaire, since it was felt that students could be more candid when confronted less directly with this issue.

The revised questionnaire was pretested in 1975, this time on 27 medical students who were completing their freshman year. This pretest was a final check on the variances and intercorrelations of the new questions not included in the first instrument. The results were very encouraging because only a few items had low variance and attitudinal items showed high correlations where expected (that is, on items measuring similar values). With added confidence from the pretest results, the long process of constructing a reliable and valid instrument to measure professional values and expectations was completed. The questionnaire was, therefore, administered in 1975 to all first-year medical students in the state of North Carolina.

Four years later, however, another questionnaire had to be devised for studying the same medical students during their senior year in order to examine changes in professional values and expectations over time. Questionnaire construction was easier this time because the same professional orientation measures were repeated in the second-wave instrument. The challenge in writing the second questionnaire was to determine and measure factors that might account for the changes in professional orientation over time. To accomplish this goal and to aid in the interpretation of the survey findings, interviews were again conducted with medical students, this time during the fall of their senior year in 1978.

In total, 18 interviews were administered—6 at each of the 3 medical schools—to the same students who would later fill out the second-wave instrument. (Interviewing only 18 of the medical students in this study was not expected to bias the final results.) Students were chosen for the interviews on the recommendation of school administrators and other students with the idea of selecting a diverse group, that is, those varying on liberalism, marital status, race, and sex.

The interviews suggested numerous factors related to students' experiences in medical school that might account for changes in orientation from first to last year. The numerous factors that might affect change (such as bad faculty role models and large debts) were listed in Chapter 2. Based on these interviews, new items were written related to students' experiences in medical school. Instead of measuring a wide variety of experiences, many items measuring a limited number of variables were preferred, so that indexes of medical school experiences could be constructed rather than relying on single items.

To pretest these new items measuring medical students' experiences, a short questionnaire was collected from an accidental sample of 21 second- and third-year medical students at Duke and the University of North Carolina in 1978. The brief pretest showed high correlation among most items intended to measure the same concept. Most pretest items were included in the second-wave questionnaire given to seniors, with only a few items omitted due to low variance. Thus, both the freshman and senior questionnaires were the products of numerous pretests and interveiws aimed at refining measurement (see Appendixes A and B).

Data Collection

The first questionnaire was distributed in the fall of 1975 to all freshman medical students in North Carolina, that is, students at Duke University School of Medicine, the University of North Carolina School of Medicine, and Bowman Gray School of Medicine. These three medical schools were chosen for this study because of their proximity and accessibility to the investigator and their likely similarity to a large proportion of medical schools in this country. The medical school at Duke is private, prestigious, and emphasizes training in research and academic medicine. Bowman Gray School of Medicine, also private, is somewhat less eminent than Duke and stresses practice more than research. The University of North Carolina Medical School is state supported and like Bowman Gray is less prestigious and less research oriented than Duke. Both Bowman Gray and the University of North Carolina draw a large proportion of their medical students from North Carolina, introducing a regional bias to the sample. Because of this regional bias, we must be cautious about generalizing the findings in this study to medical students nationwide.

Questionnaires were distributed during freshman orientation at the three medical schools. The author went to each orientation to request an immediate response to the questionnaire and to explain the purpose of the project in general terms. Students were promised anonymity and feedback on the results of the study. At all schools, a school administrator also encouraged participation in the study, although it was made clear that the study was not sponsored by the school. Follow-up letters reminding students to fill out the questionnaire were sent a few days after orientation. Follow-up was a little more difficult at Bowman Gray since that school requested that names be omitted from the questionnaire.

Of the 353 entering students at all schools, 92 percent returned the questionnaire. The returned questionnaires represented virtually the total population of first-year medical students in 1975 in the state of North Carolina. The investigator's presence at freshman orientation, the freshmen's apparent enthusiasm at beginning medical school, the emphasis on quickly returning the questionnaire, and the intensive follow-up appear to account for the high response rate during the freshman year.

To examine changes over time, the author distributed a second questionnaire to the same medical students during their senior year from late fall through early winter 1978/79. Questionnaires were mailed to students at Duke and the University of North Carolina, since that was the only way to contact students at these schools. Letters to remind these students to fill out the questionnaire were mailed a few weeks later and numerous phone calls were made to encourage participation. Most students expressed interest in the research and remembered the investigator from freshman orientation. Delayed responses seemed to be a result of time pressures; very few students actually refused to participate. New questionnaires were sent to all nonrespondents after their Christmas break.

At Bowman Gray, the researcher was fortunate to be given a time when most students would be present to distribute the questionnaire. The students filled out the instrument while the researcher waited. For those students who were absent that day, a notice was posted about the study. No other follow-up procedures were possible because names were again not allowed on the questionnaires at that school.

Some decisions had to be made about who was eligible to fill out the second-wave questionnaire since some students in the original 1975 entering classes had dropped back a year or two, had excelled and just graduated, or had entered the M.D./Ph.D. program (only at Duke) and thus had completed only two or three years of medical school. From the original study population, the author decided to include the few who had dropped back to the third but not second year of medical school, those who had graduated, and those who were in the combined-degree program. * Of those returning both freshman and senior questionnaires, only 2 percent were in their third year, 4 percent had graduated, and 4 percent were in the combined-degree program. An analysis of variance showed no statistically significant differences on professional orientation between these three subgroups and the other students, except that the combined-degree students were less interested in primary-care medicine. This was not surprising since the M.D./Ph.D. program was designed for those interested in academic medicine and research. Therefore, the investigator did not differentiate between these categories of students in the data analysis because the vast majority of students had followed the regular career path; not following it did not seem to make much difference in terms of professional values. As a general rule, students who did not start medical school with the original entering class in 1975, but were seniors during the second wave of data collection, were not sent the questionnaire.

The return rate for the second-wave questionnaire was also quite high despite the response problems with mailed questionnaires and the difficulties with contacting students who had graduated. Of the 341 medical students still available in 1978 at the three schools (only eight had dropped out or transferred and four had dropped back to the second year), 87 percent returned the questionnaire. The persistent phone calls and the personal contact with students four years earlier probably contributed greatly to the enthusiastic response.

The return rates for the first- and second-wave questionnaires at each school in total and by sex are given in Table 3.1. There are no statistically significant differences between the return rates of men and women overall or within schools on either questionnaire. Variations on return rates between schools are not different from chance except on the first-wave questionnaire where Bowman Gray students were less likely to return the instrument than students at the University of North Carolina. The follow-up difficulty at Bowman Gray (where no names were allowed on questionnaires) probably accounts for the lower response rate at that school in 1975. These school variations are most likely unimportant considering the high response at all three institutions.

----

*Because Duke students do clinical rotations in their second year of medical school, it was decided that the M.D./Ph.D. students had at least that important experience. To eliminate these students would have biased the sample against those interested in research because those working for both clinical and academic degrees usually pursue careers in academic medicine.

TABLE 3.1

Return Rates for the First- and Second-Wave Questionnaires by School and by Sex

School	First Wave, 1975						Second Wave, 1978					
	Male		Female		Total		Male		Female		Total	
	Per-cent	Num-ber	Per-cent	Num-ber	Per-cent	Num-ber	Per-cent	Num-ber	Per-cent	Num-ber	Per-cent	Num-ber
Duke	91	80	89	35	90	115	83	78	88	33	85	111
North Carolina	96	108	100	32	97	140	89	105	90	29	89	134
Bowman Gray	88	76	86	22	88	98	84	75	95	21	86	96
Total	92	264	92	89	92	353	86	258	90	83	87	341

Note: The return rates for the first-wave questionnaire are based on the number of entering freshmen in each of the table categories. These numbers may vary from published figures because of students dropping out early, entering late, or repeating the first year. The return rates for the second-wave questionnaire are based on the number of entering freshmen in each table category minus those who dropped out, transferred, or dropped back to their second year of medical school. Chi-square was computed to test for significant differences at the .05 level on return rates for each questionnaire by sex and by school.

54

TABLE 3.2

Percentage of Medical Students Returning Both Questionnaires by
Sex and School

School	Male		Female		Total	
	Percent	Number	Percent	Number	Percent	Number
Duke	78	78	85	33	80	111
North Carolina	88	105	90	29	88	134
Bowman Gray	72	75	86	21	75	96
Total	80	258	87	83	82	341

Note: The return rates are based on the number of students in
each category that could have answered both questionnaires, that is,
entering freshmen minus those who dropped out, transferred, or
dropped back to their second year of medical school.

Since the bulk of the data analysis examines changes in medical
students' professional values over time, the first- and second-wave
questionnaires were matched for each student. Although no names
were on the Bowman Gray questionnaires, students' responses from
their freshman year were paired with their senior-year answers based
on birth date and other identifying background information. Although
some of the analysis could have been done on all those who answered
the first wave and all those answering the second wave, some results
would have included more students than others. In other words, some
data analyses would have reported information only on those who answered both questionnaires and some would have included the larger
group who either responded to one or both instruments. In order to
make all data analyses consistent and to ensure valid comparison
groups, all findings were calculated on the subgroup of students
(279) who answered both freshman and senior questionnaires unless
otherwise indicated. For the most part, analyzing this subset of
students does not alter the results. Thus, 47 students who responded
to the first questionnaire but not the second and 18 students who answered only the second instrument have been omitted from data analyses, unless otherwise indicated.

Table 3.2 shows the return rates at each school in total and by sex for those returning both freshman and senior questionnaires. There are no statistically significant sex differences overall or within schools on returning both questionnaires, although women tend toward slightly greater participation. Again, Bowman Gray has a somewhat lower return rate owing to their lower response on the first instrument and to their larger proportion of students returning only one questionnaire. Because of the enthusiastic response of most medical students, the subset of students answering both questionnaires is still a quite high proportion (82 percent) of the students who both began medical school in North Carolina in 1975 and were in the study population in 1978.[1] Although the sample represents virtually the total population of students in North Carolina, inferential statistics are computed in most data analyses as a nonsubjective method for deciding whether the data exhibit random or systematic variation.

MEASUREMENT

Because this research presents a new conceptualization of professional values and expectations, a detailed account of how these variables have been measured is given next. In addition, the measurement of explanatory variables that may account for why the sexes differ in professional orientation or why changes in orientation occur over time is also detailed. Explanatory variables include measures of social background attributes, personality and political outlook characteristics, and reactions to a variety of medical school experiences.

Professional Values and Expectations

As mentioned previously, numerous questions were written to measure each of the professional orientations listed in Chapter 1. Most questions concerning professional values were scaled on a five-point continuum including agree strongly, agree somewhat, neutral opinion, disagree somewhat, and disagree strongly. The neutral category facilitated the detection of nonsalient issues by not forcing students to select an opinion. Most items concerning professional expectations were scaled on a four-point continuum including very likely, somewhat likely, somewhat unlikely, and very unlikely.

Since indexes (measures composed of two or more questionnaire items) tend to be more reliable than single-item measures, the author wanted to create indexes of professional orientations rather than rely on responses to individual questions. In order to construct meaningful indexes, a systematic method was needed for summarizing the numerous correlations among items measuring professional values and expectations. Factor analysis was the technique employed, because it is designed to reduce many variables to fewer underlying unities or factors.[2]

Items tapping each of the professional values and expectations were expected to cluster into distinct factors. Before actually doing the factor analysis, a factor solution was hypothesized. As predicted, the hypothesized theoretical solution and the actual factor solution were similar. In the few cases where the two solutions differed, theoretical considerations guided the construction of indexes. The factor solution was therefore treated as support for the underlying hypothesized constructs rather than as an exploratory method for finding attitudinal dimensions.

With so many professional orientation items (74 in all), one factor analysis was not feasible. Therefore, professional orientation items were divided into the following three general groupings for factoring: 36 value items concerning the profession and the practice of medicine, 23 expectation items concerning the kind of physician the student planned to be, and 15 value and expectation items concerning influences on the student's choice of medicine as a career.* These three groups tapped distinct but broad substantive areas. They were selected as a means of controlling for methods variance so that questions stated in the first person were factored discretely from those stated in the third person, since these groups tend to cluster separately. The professional orientation items have been divided into three domains for convenience, thus these groups do not reflect any theoretical classification of professional values and expectations. Furthermore, the factor analysis was performed on data from all the freshman questionnaires (326 cases) because at the time of the analysis only first-wave data were available.

The factor loadings for the three domains showed a fairly distinct factor structure with a diverse set of factors emerging. The factor analysis of the 36 items concerning the profession and the practice of medicine yielded 10 factors with eigenvalues above one.[3] This

---

*The numbers next to items in the three domains for factoring that follow are found on the freshman questionnaire in Appendix A. The 36 value items concerning the profession and the practice of medicine are questions 43, 46, 47(1-4, 6-16, 18-21, 23, 25, 26, 30-39, 42, 43). The 23 expectation items concerning the kind of physician the student plans to be are questions 31(1-11), 34, 35, 36, 38, 47(5, 17, 22, 24, 28, 29, 40, 41). The 15 value and expectation items concerning influences on the student's choice of medicine as a career are questions 28(1-15).

TABLE 3.3

Means and Standard Deviations for Indexes and for Items in Measures concerning the Doctor/Patient Relationship, with Inter-Item Correlations for Each Index, in Freshman Year

Index and Item	Mean	Standard Deviation	Range of Value	Inter-Item Correlation, Item Number		
				2	3	4
Important to provide health information to patients	3.29	0.78	1-5			
1. Nurses should have a good deal of latitude in giving information to patients (agree = high)	2.84	1.08	1-5	.26	.26	.29
2. Information about diagnosis and treatment should be given to patients so they can better evaluate the physician's competence (agree = high)	3.59	1.13	1-5	—	.21	.27
3. The patient should be told everything concerning his diagnosis and possible treatment(s) (agree = high)	3.33	1.23	1-5		—	.25
4. A patient should have access to his or her own medical records (agree = high)	3.39	1.29	1-5			—
Patients should not have absolute confidence in physicians' judgments	2.80	1.08	1-5			
1. It is always inappropriate for a physician to make critical remarks to a patient concerning another physician (disagree = high)	2.48	1.28	1-5	.40		
2. Patients should have absolute confidence in the judgments of physicians (disagree = high)	3.11	1.30	1-5	—		

58

Social and psychological factors, including empathy, are important in health care

	Mean	SD	Range		
Social and psychological factors, including empathy, are important in health care	4.29	0.57	1-5		
1. Medical training must emphasize learning how to deal with the social and psychological problems of patients as much as learning medical facts (agree = high)	4.78	0.51	1-5	.16	.18
2. Physicians realistically cannot be very empathetic with their patients; it is hard enough to do the technical aspects of their job well (disagree = high)	4.28	0.84	1-5	—	.24
3. It is more important for a physician to have extensive knowledge of medical facts than an ability to establish rapport with patients (disagree = high)	3.82	1.08	1-5		
Chose medicine in order to help people*	3.35	0.58	1-4		—
1. The chance to make a real contribution to mankind (important = high)	3.14	0.84	1-4	.20	.51
2. It gives me an opportunity to work with people rather than things (important = high)	3.46	0.74	1-4	—	.51
3. Gives me the opportunity to help others (important = high)	3.46	0.69	1-4		—

*The freshman questionnaire asked students, "How important were the following factors in influencing your choice of medicine as a career?" The senior instrument asked students, "How important are the following factors to you as you think about your career in medicine?"

Note: Data are based on freshman responses. All data on items are calculated on approximately 326 cases (all those responding to the first questionnaire minus nonrespondents). All data on indexes are based on exactly 326 cases, because nonrespondents are coded to the mean on each item. All items are coded in the same attitudinal direction as indicated in parentheses so that all correlations are positive and means are consistent with the index label. All correlations are significant at the .01 level.

TABLE 3.4

Means and Standard Deviations for Indexes and for Items in Measures concerning Political and Economic Change in the Medical Profession, with Inter-Item Correlations for Each Index, in Freshman Year

Index and Item	Mean	Standard Deviation	Range of Value	Inter-Item Correlation, Item Number			
				2	3	4	5
Profession's control over health should be reduced through government intervention and socialized medicine	2.96	1.03	1-5				
1. It is very important to protect the autonomy of the medical profession against government intervention (disagree = high)	2.54	1.23	1-5	.64	.35	.71	.59
2. I am opposed to a system of socialized medicine in this country (disagree = high)	2.94	1.45	1-5	—	.35	.66	.57
3. Review committees should be established by the federal government to insure that physicians do not overcharge for their services (agree = high)	3.44	1.26	1-5		—	.41	.34
4. I feel that the medical profession should keep their control over all aspects of the profession, rather than have government intervention (disagree = high)	2.85	1.33	1-5			—	.61
5. Generally, I am opposed to government intervention and control in order to solve social problems (disagree = high)	3.04	1.27	1-5				—
Physicians' status and financial rewards need to be lowered	3.06	0.85	1-5				
1. How much money a year do you think a physician working 40 hours a week should make? (small amount = high)[a]	3.20	1.32	1-7	.51	.33	.33	
2. Because physicians undergo long and expensive training, they deserve the income they make (disagree = high)	2.56	1.26	1-5	—	.44	.39	

	Mean	S.D.	Range			
3. Physicians deserve to earn more money than other people in this society (disagree = high)	3.34	1.21	1-5		—	.34
4. Prestige distinctions between nurses and physicians should <u>not</u> be reduced (disagree = high)	3.30	1.16	1-5			—
High status and income were important in career selection[b]	1.94	0.60	1-4			
1. The chance to live a financially secure and prosperous life (important = high)	2.21	0.76	1-4	.45	.26	.31
2. The chance to gain status and prestige with my colleagues and in the community (important = high)	1.94	0.80	1-4	—	.45	.62
3. Medicine is (was) seen as a glamorous field (important = high)	1.57	0.76	1-4	.45	—	.45
4. The chance to gain respect from others (important = high)	2.01	0.84	1-4			—
Expect to work for political and social change in medicine	2.20	0.75	1-4			
1. Using medicine to change society or the medical system (important = high)	1.99	0.99	1-4		.29	.55
2. Public health medicine (likely = high)	2.32	0.89	1-4		—	.38
3. Physician working for political and social change in medicine (likely = high)	2.27	1.01	1-4			—

aThe remainder of the question reads (1) under $15,000, (2) $15,001 to $20,000, (3) $20,001 to $25,000, (4) $25,001 to $30,000, (5) $30,001 to $40,000, (6) $40,001 to $50,000, (7) over $50,000. These responses were recoded for the index from one to five as follows: (1) over $50,000, (2) $40,001 to $50,000, (3) $30,001 to $40,000, (4) $20,001 to $30,000, and (5) under $20,000. The mean on this recoded item is 3.04 with a standard deviation of 1.07.

bThe freshman questionnaire asked students, "How important were the following factors in influencing your choice of medicine as a career?" The senior instrument asked students, "How important are the following factors to you as you think about your career in medicine?"

<u>Note</u>: Data are based on freshmen responses. All data on items are calculated on approximately 326 cases (all those responding to the first questionnaire minus nonrespondents). All data on indexes are based on exactly 326 cases because nonrespondents are coded to the mean on each item. All items are coded in the same attitudinal direction as indicated in parentheses so that all correlations are positive and means are consistent with the index label. All correlations are significant at the .01 level.

TABLE 3.5

Means and Standard Deviations for Indexes and for Items in Measures concerning the Treatment of Women Physicians and Patients, with Inter-Item Correlations for Each Index, in Freshman Year

Index and Item	Mean	Standard Deviation	Range of Value	Inter-Item Correlation, Item Number		
				2	3	4
There is professional and public prejudice against women physicians	2.97	0.91	1-5			
1. Medical school and the medical profession are harder for a woman than a man because many students and professors are prejudiced against women (agree = high)	2.71	1.15	1-5	.43		
2. Medical school and the medical profession are harder for a woman than a man because many patients are prejudiced against women doctors (agree = high)	3.22	1.02	1-5	—		
There is pressure on women physicians to choose certain fields, such as pediatrics	3.19	0.93	1-5			
1. The medical profession places pressure on women to specialize in certain fields of medicine, like pediatrics (agree = high)	3.17	1.04	1-5	.62		
2. Women medical students are not discouraged from specializing in certain fields of medicine, like surgery (disagree = high)	3.21	1.03	1-5	—		
There is a need for more women physicians in this country	3.97	0.92	1-5			
1. It would be damaging to the profession of medicine if half the students admitted to medical schools were women (disagree = high)	4.05	1.17	1-5	.50		
2. We definitely need more women physicians in this country (agree = high)	3.90	0.98	1-5	—		
Physicians generally treat women patients in a patronizing and prejudicial way	3.03	0.72	1-5			
1. Gynecologists generally treat female patients with respect and concern (disagree = high)	2.54	1.07	1-5	.28	.47	.46
2. Male physicians tend to treat female patients in a more patronizing way then they treat male patients (agree = high)	3.18	0.96	1-5	—	.36	.30
3. Generally, male physicians are as sensitive as they should be to the needs of female patients (disagree = high)	3.20	0.99	1-5		—	.50
4. Gynecologists generally have an accurate view of female sexuality (disagree = high)	3.20	0.88	1-5			—

Note: Data are based on freshmen responses. All data on items are calculated on approximately 326 cases (all those responding to the first questionnaire minus nonrespondents). All data on indexes are based on exactly 326 cases, because nonrespondents are coded to the mean on each item. All items are coded in the same attitudinal direction as indicated in parentheses so that all correlations are positive and means are consistent with the index label. All correlations are significant at the .01 level.

TABLE 3.6

Means and Standard Deviations for Indexes and for Items in Measures concerning Physician Maldistribution, with Inter-Item Correlations for Each Index, in Freshman Year

Index and Item	Mean	Standard Deviation	Range of Value	Inter-Item Correlation, Item Number		
				2	3	4
Expect to practice primary-care medicine	3.85	1.13	1-5			
1. Primary-care physician (general practice) (likely = high)[a]	3.10	0.98	1-4	.68		
2. I feel a great personal commitment to primary-care medicine (agree = high)	3.86	1.10	1-5	—		
Committed to choosing a specialty and geographic area that need physicians	3.63	1.06	1-5			
1. If I had to choose between the following two practices, I'd choose:[b]	1.65	0.48	1-2	.51	.51	.36
2. I am strongly committed to locating my practice in an area of the country that needs physicians (agree = high)	3.57	1.18	1-5	—	.72	.66
3. I do not plan to practice in a medically deprived area (disagree = high)	3.69	1.08	1-5		—	.54
4. I am strongly committed to choosing a field of medicine where there is great medical need (agree = high)	3.65	1.13	1-5			—

[a] Primary care refers to physicians of first contact offering a relatively full scope of services. For example, family practitioners, general pediatricians, general internists, and gynecologists who do little or no surgery are primary-care physicians. This item originally ranged from one to four, but it has been recoded for the index as follows: (1) very unlikely, (2) somewhat unlikely, (4) somewhat likely, and (5) very likely. The mean on this recoded item is 3.84 with a standard deviation of 1.37.

[b] The remainder of the question reads as follows:

1. A practice in an intellectually stimulating environment but where the need for another physician was not great.
2. A practice in an area with little intellectual stimulation but where a physician was very much needed. (response two = high)

This item was recoded for the index by changing two to five. The mean on this recoded item is 3.61 with a standard deviation of 1.91.

Note: Data are based on freshmen responses. All data on items are calculated on approximately 326 cases (all those responding to the first questionnaire minus nonrespondents). All data on indexes are based on exactly 326 cases, because nonrespondents are coded to the mean on each item. All items are coded in the same attitudinal direction as indicated in parentheses so that all correlations are positive and means are consistent with the index label. All correlations are significant at the .01 level.

explained 58 percent of the total variance in the matrix. The 23 items pertaining to career expectations formed 7 factors with eigenvalues above one; this explained 64 percent of the total variance. Finally, the factoring of the 15 items referring to career influences yielded 5 factors with eigenvalues above one; this explained 61 percent of the total variance in the matrix. It is not surprising that numerous factors with eigenvalues above one were found considering the large number of items and the broad range of issues covered within these domains.

The factor-loadings matrix for each of the three domains are not given here since these weights were not used in the creation of indexes of professional orientation. [4] In all cases, items were weighted equally in the formation of indexes, and a mean score on each index was computed for each respondent. There were so little missing data that all nonresponses were coded to the mean on each item. Indexes ranged in scores from either one to five or one to four corresponding to the number of possible responses to the questionnaire items in each index. Therefore, indexes containing items with a neutral category ranged from one to five; all others ranged from one to four.

Index construction followed the factor solution very closely, so that items loading .40 or greater were included in an index. In a few cases where items loaded on two factors, the item was included in the index corresponding to its highest factor loading. Deviations from the factor solution were made for theoretical reasons, so that the indexes made theoretical as well as statistical sense.

Tables 3.3 to 3.6 give the exact wording of items in each professional orientation index with inter-item correlations and means and standard deviations for each item. The indexes in these tables are organized by health problem areas, that is, the doctor/patient relationship, the need for political and economic change in the medical profession, the treatment of women physicians and patients, and physician maldistribution. All items in Tables 3.3 to 3.6 are coded so that a high number refers to high agreement or support of a particular orientation as stated in the index label. Since all items are coded in the same attitudinal direction as the index labels (indicated in parentheses), the means do not always correspond to the exact wording of the questionnaire item. Scoring high on an index usually indicates holding values and expectations considered beneficial for health care. * Since the factor analysis was originally performed on data from the first-wave questionnaire, the data in Tables 3.3 to 3.6

---

*The index measuring the importance of high status and income in career selection is an exception to the rule that scoring high on an index indicates holding values beneficial for health care.

are based on those who responded to the first instrument (326 cases minus missing data).

Tables 3.3 to 3.6 show generally moderate to high correlations among items in each professional orientation index. The index concerning the importance of social and psychological factors in health care is an exception to this trend. The low inter-item correlations are due in part to the low variance on some of the items in this index. Few students deny the importance of learning how to deal with patients' social and psychological problems.

Apart from the indexes listed in Tables 3.3 to 3.6, a few single-item measures of professional orientation have also been examined in this study, either because they were considered theoretically separate from the factors on which they loaded or they did not load on any factors. Included are the following items relating to political and economic issues in medicine:

1. What percentage of your time do you expect to do volunteer work as a physician? * (Responses ranged from 0 to 80 percent.)

2. We need to change the health-care system in this country so that drug companies, insurance companies, and hospitals cannot make profits from health care. (Responses ranged from one to five on a disagree-to-agree scale.)

3. Would you be in favor of a National Service Corps for physicians in which every physician, male or female, would have to serve one or two years in a medically deprived area in order to obtain a permanent license? (Responses ranged from one to three and included no; yes, only if medical education is paid for by the government; and yes.)

The other two single-item professional orientation measures included in this study asked students to think about the kind of physician they will most likely be. Ranging from one to four on a very unlikely to very likely scale, these items concern the problem of geographic maldistribution of physicians, that is, planning a rural practice and planning to be an inner-city physician taking care of low-income minority groups.

Table 3.7 shows the matrix of intercorrelations among all the professional orientation indexes and single-item measures during the first and the last year of medical school for all those who answered both questionnaires. Cronbach's alpha,[5] an internal consistency re-

---

*Volunteer work includes working in a free clinic and giving free care to those who cannot pay; it does not include time spent with patients who do not pay their bills or professional-courtesy patients.

TABLE 3.7

Intercorrelations of Professional Orientation Indexes and Single-Item Measures for Medical Students' Freshman Year (Upper Half of Matrix) and Senior Year (Lower Half of Matrix)

Problem Area and Variable	1	2	3	4	5	6	7	8	9	10	11	12	13	14	15	16	17	18	19
Doctor/patient relationship																			
1. Give health information	—	.14	.06	-.04	.26	.24	.21	.30	-.10	.28	.12	.12	.13	.29	.18	.06	.02	.12	.05
2. Be critical of doctors	.29	—	-.03	-.08	.25	-.03	-.00	.31	-.21	.15	.12	.18	.07	.11	.27	.00	.07	.08	.04
3. Social/psychological important	.24	.09	—	.21	.03	.13	.06	.14	-.07	.09	.08	.11	.15	.14	.25	.23	.05	.09	.07
4. Helping people important	.04	-.01	.20	—	.04	.05	-.05	.04	.11	.13	.16	-.07	.00	.04	.03	.38	.17	.11	.31
Political and economic change																			
5. Reduce profession's control	.25	.35	.17	.02	—	.33	.28	.50	-.18	.45	.19	.14	.14	.34	.27	-.02	.05	.28	.11
6. Favor National Service Corps	.18	.17	.13	.08	.28	—	.14	.21	-.19	.18	.15	-.06	.09	.23	.16	.03	-.04	.11	.06
7. No profits in health care	.14	.08	.14	.17	.38	.18	—	.30	-.12	.23	.17	.07	.09	.21	.30	-.02	-.01	.14	-.01
8. Lower doctor's income	.26	.38	.21	.11	.54	.29	.31	—	-.39	.40	.25	.16	.19	.38	.37	.03	.07	.27	.18
9. Money/status are important	-.06	-.18	-.06	-.01	-.21	-.11	-.21	-.39	—	-.04	-.08	-.05	.04	-.11	-.21	-.05	-.09	-.09	-.14
10. Work for political change	.24	.24	.22	.28	.40	.24	.32	.39	-.17	—	.31	.14	.16	.27	.25	.12	.10	.34	.24
11. Plan volunteer work	.04	.13	.08	.30	.10	.18	.22	.20	-.05	.24	—	.07	.02	.12	.14	.15	.16	.34	.29
Women physicians and patients																			
12. Bias toward women doctors	.12	.12	.01	.06	.10	.01	.13	.17	-.05	.15	.03	—	.38	.27	.35	-.03	.00	.04	.01
13. Specialty choice pressure	.06	.18	-.00	.02	.13	.12	.14	.15	-.03	.13	.02	.44	—	.25	.40	.01	.00	.08	.02
14. Need more women doctors	.34	.35	.27	.05	.35	.27	.19	.39	-.16	.25	-.01	.31	.32	—	.35	-.02	-.03	.22	.02
15. Bias toward women patients	.18	.28	.14	-.00	.36	.09	.22	.28	-.12	.26	.01	.38	.44	.50	—	.11	.02	.20	.07
Physician maldistribution																			
16. Plan primary-care medicine	.06	.01	.22	.40	.09	.01	.08	.16	-.12	.27	.18	-.02	.04	.07	.08	—	.53	.11	.55
17. Plan rural practice	.02	.05	.12	.27	.01	.07	.02	.17	-.09	.17	.30	-.07	-.06	-.04	-.04	.60	—	.13	.65
18. Plan inner-city practice	.10	.19	.14	.18	.35	.15	.26	.23	-.11	.46	.25	.11	.12	.18	.17	.16	.07	—	.26
19. Committed to patient need	.02	.01	.22	.39	.08	.07	.14	.23	-.10	.28	.34	-.06	-.04	.01	-.02	.65	.70	.22	—

Note: Measures 6, 7, 11, 17, and 18 are single items. All others are indexes composed of two or more variables. Data are based on all students who responded to both the freshman- and senior-year questionnaires. Thus, correlations are based on 279 cases with the exception of single-item measures, which are calculated on slightly fewer cases due to nonresponses. All correlations of about .11 and higher are significant at the .05 probability level.

66

TABLE 3.8

Reliabilities (Cronbach's Alpha) of Professional Orientation Indexes Measured in the
Freshman and Senior Year
(for those students who returned both questionnaires, N = 279)

	Reliability (Cronbach's Alpha)	
Problem Area and Variable	Freshman Year	Senior Year

Doctor/patient relationship

1. Important to provide health information to patients	.60	.52
2. Patients should not have absolute confidence in physicians' judgments.	.59	.57
3. Social and psychological factors, including empathy, are important in health care	.40	.36
4. Chose medicine in order to help people (helping people is important part of medical career)*	.67	.73

Political and economic change in the profession

5. Profession's control over health should be reduced through government intervention and socialized medicine	.84	.83
6. Physicians' status and financial rewards need to be lowered	.68	.72
7. High status and income were important in career selection (high status and income are important part of medical career) *	.74	.76
8. Expect to work for political and social change in medicine	.67	.73

Treatment of women physicians and patients

9. There is pressure on women physicians to choose certain fields, such as pediatrics	.73	.76
10. There is professional and public prejudice against women physicians	.59	.59
11. There is a need for more women physicians in this country	.68	.68
12. Physicians generally treat women patients in a patronizing and prejudicial way	.72	.80

Physician maldistribution

13. Expect to practice primary-care medicine	.82	.89
14. Committed to choosing a specialty and geographic area that need physicians	.82	.87

*Approximate wording on freshman questionnaire shown with approximate
wording on senior questionnaire in parentheses.

liability measure, is shown in Table 3.8 for professional orientation indexes measured during freshman and senior years. The reliability measure is a summary of the inter-item correlations weighted by the numbers of items. As the inter-item correlations and the number of items increase so does the calculated alpha.

As expected, given the orthogonal (uncorrelated) factor solution, Table 3.7 shows that index score correlations are fairly low in both first and last years. Especially low correlations are shown between measures intended to differ conceptually. Treating coefficient alpha as a measure of internal consistency, Tables 3.7 and 3.8 show that each index correlates more highly with itself than with any other index or single-item measure in both freshman and senior years. The general pattern of low correlations between indexes and the substantial reliability coefficients lend both discriminant and convergent validation to the professional orientation measures. [6] Where indexes do tend to correlate, the clusters substantiate the theoretical grouping of orientations into the four health-care problem areas. The data provide strong empirical support for the theoretical conception of professional values and expectations presented in this report.

A second factor analysis based on professional orientations measured in the senior year confirmed the original factor structure on first-year responses with inter-item correlations similar to those calculated the first year. As indicated by the substantial senior-year reliabilities in Table 3.8, moderate to high correlations were found among most professional orientation items grouped into indexes. In fact, reliabilities on professional orientations measured in the senior year tended to be slightly higher than those calculated on freshman-year responses. The exceptions to this trend were on indexes concerning the importance of providing health information to patients and of paying attention to social and psychological factors in health care. On these measures the reliabilities tended to decrease slightly from freshman to senior year. Most professional orientation indexes, however, showed substantial internal consistency in both years of measurement, and therefore we can be fairly confident in the reliability of most of these measures.

Explanatory Variables

Social Background Attributes

In order to account for the initial sex differences in professional orientations or the changes in orientations over time, the researchers' first step was to determine if social background characteristics had an explanatory role. Therefore, numerous social background items were included on both freshman and senior questionnaires. Because the measurement of most social background variables is self-explanatory, the following discussion is fairly brief. Items are coded so that a low number indicates low on interval measures.

The following social background characteristics have been included in this study: medical school attending (Duke, University of North Carolina, or Bowman Gray), freshman- and senior-year martial status (single or married, other coded missing), race (white or black, other coded missing), sex, senior-year parental status (having children), age, father's education, father's socioeconomic status (index scores based on 1960 census classifications),[7] age decided to study medicine, presence of physicians in one's family, number of physicians in one's family, presence of a physician father, presence of physician friends, urban/rural background,* religion (Protestant, Catholic, Jewish, and none), religiosity in freshman year (four-point scale ranging from religion has no importance in one's life to very much importance), and debts expected upon completion of training.

Personality and Political Outlook

In addition to examining whether background variables accounted for the initial sex differences in professional orientations, the potential explanatory role of personality and general political outlook variables also has been analyzed. In other words, the data analysis will determine if the sex differences on professional orientations upon entrance to school reflect personality and political outlook differences between men and women. The personality attributes measured on the freshman questionnaire include nurturance, dominance, cynicism, and competitiveness.†

Measures of nurturance and dominance have been adapted from the Personality Research Form,[8] an inventory chosen because it is designed for highly educated populations and seems to have face validity. Nurturance is defined as sympathetic, maternal, helpful, caring, and supporting. Dominance is described as controlling, governing, influential, forceful, assertive, and powerful.

The dominance and nurturance personality scales in the Personality Research Form are each composed of 20 items. Owing to problems of questionnaire length, however, the researcher randomly

---

*Urban/rural background variables are defined as follows: rural (under 2,500 population), small city or town (2,500 to less than 50,000), suburb of a small or medium city, medium city (50,000 to 250,000), suburb of a large city, and large city (over 250,000).

† Cynicism and competitiveness were measured on the senior questionnaire as well as the freshman instrument.

selected only 15 of the nurturance questions and 10 of the dominance items for the freshman questionnaire. * The length for each personality measure was chosen by using the Spearman-Brown prophecy formula to ensure adequate reliability (an estimated alpha coefficient greater than .65).[9]

To ensure sufficient variance on the personality measures, these items were scaled to four categories of agree to disagree, instead of the two categories used in the Personality Research Form. The freshman questionnaire in Appendix A shows the exact wording of the items in the nurturance and dominance scales. † In creating indexes of personality, all items were weighted equally and a mean score from one to four was computed for each index; higher scores indicated more dominance and nurturance. Since nonresponse was extremely low, all missing values were coded to the grand mean corresponding to each item in creating index scores. The computed Cronbach's alpha coefficients of scale reliability for the 15-item nurturance measure and the 10-item dominance scale were .75 and .72, respectively.

A measure of cynicism also has been included as an explanatory personality variable, since an implicit assumption of much research is that cynicism affects one's professional values. Thus, if the sexes vary in their degree of cynicism, this might account for some initial sex differences in professional orientations. A five-item cynical realism personality measure is included in both questionnaires.[10] Cynicism as measured here refers to an attitude reflecting the belief that most people try to use others to get ahead in life. ‡ Like the other personality measures, the five items tapping cynicism were equally weighted and a mean score from one to four was computed for each respondent; higher scores indicated greater cynicism. The computed reliability for the cynicism scale was .61, slightly lower than that reported previously.[11]

Only one item has been included on the questionnaire to measure competitiveness, another personality attribute that might explain some

---

*It would have been preferable to select those statements with the highest inter-item or item-to-total correlations from the two personality inventories; however, this information was not readily available.

† The nurturance questions on the freshman questionnaire are items 30(3, 4, 5, 8, 12, 13, 17, 18, 20, 22, 24, 26, 28, 29, 30). The dominance questions are items 30(1, 2, 7, 9, 10, 14, 16, 19, 23, 25).

‡ The exact wording of items measuring cynicism is shown as follows on the freshman questionnaire in Appendix A: questions 30(6, 11, 15, 21, 27).

TABLE 3.9

Means, Standard Deviations, and Intercorrelations of Personality
and Political Outlook Measures in Freshman Year
(index reliabilities—Cronbach's alpha—reported on the diagonal of
the matrix)

Variable	1	2	3	4	5	Mean	Standard Deviation
1. Nurturance	(.75)	.12	-.37	-.02	.02	3.03	0.33
2. Dominance		(.72)	.03	.31	.01	2.74	0.41
3. Cynicism			(.61)	.02	-.07	1.60	0.42
4. Competitive-ness				(—)	-.10	2.62	1.17
5. Political liberalism					(—)	3.39	0.79

Note: All data are based on 279 cases, those who answered
both freshman and senior questionnaires, except data on "competitiveness" and "political liberalism," which are calculated on 276 and 266
cases, respectively, because of nonresponses. Competitiveness and
political liberalism are single-item measures ranging from one to
five. All other measures are indexes ranging from one to four. All
correlations of about .11 and higher are significant at the .05 probability level.

of the initial sex differences on professional orientations. This item,
ranging from one to five on an agreement scale that includes a neutral
category, reads as follows: "I dislike competition with other people
when the stakes are high." Agreeing with this statement indicates a
low score on competitiveness. Because other personality characteristics were expected to be more important explanatory variables than
competitiveness and to avoid an excessively long questionnaire, only
one item measuring competitiveness was included.

In addition to the personality measures, the respondent's general political orientation was also expected to be an important variable accounting for the initial sex differences on professional orientations. To measure political outlook students were asked, "Where
would you place yourself in terms of a general political outlook?" The
following responses were coded from one to five: radical right, con-

servative, middle of the road, liberal, and radical left. A higher number indicated greater liberalism.

Table 3.9 shows the means, standard deviations, and intercorrelations of political outlook and personality variables, with index reliabilities reported on the diagonal of the matrix. These variables show a general pattern of high internal consistency with low between-measure correlations. The correlations that do occur are in expected directions so that cynicism is negatively related to nurturance, and dominance is positively related to competitiveness. *

Experiences in Medical School

One of the main goals of this research was to determine why changes in students' values occur from freshman to senior year. Of particular interest was the role, if any, of the medical school in bringing about changes in professional orientations. Therefore, to explain changes in professional orientations over time, the author focused mainly on factors related to students' experiences in medical school. The measurement of these factors will be detailed next.

The questionnaire distributed during students' senior year contained 33 questions related to students' experiences in medical school.† Factor analysis was used to summarize the numerous correlations among these items and thus aided in the creation of indexes. Although index construction followed the factor solution quite closely, theoretical considerations entered into index construction decisions as well. For example, items pertaining to how doctors treat both patients and students loaded on the same factor but were divided into separate student and patient treatment indexes, because they were considered theoretically distinct issues.

The factor analysis of the 33 items concerning experiences in medical school yielded 10 factors with eigenvalues above 1, which explained 64 percent of the total variance in the matrix. The large number of items and the broad range of issues covered resulted in the emergence of this large and diverse set of factors.

---

*One of the professional values (the importance of high status and income in career selection) was also included in the analysis explaining initial sex differences in professional orientations. The measurement of this variable was described previously with professional values and expectations.

† The following 33 questions measuring students' experiences in medical school were on the questionnaire administered during students' senior year: questions 30, 31, 32, 33, 41, 42, 43, 44, 45(4, 10, 16, 24, 28, 34, 46), 47(1-3), 49(1-6), 50(1-6).

Most indexes were constructed so that they included items that had factor loadings of at least .40. Based primarily on the factor analysis, seven of the school-experiences items were constructed. In all cases, items were weighted equally in the formation of indexes, and a mean score of each index was computed for each respondent. The small number of missing cases were assigned the mean on each item. Indexes ranged in value from one to four or one to five corresponding to the number of possible responses on the items in each index. Where indexes contained items with a different number of response categories, the items with fewer categories were recoded so they would be consistent with the items having a larger range of possible responses.

Table 3.10 gives the exact wording of items that were grouped into indexes of school experiences with inter-item correlations for each index and means and standard deviations for items and indexes. All items are coded so that a low number refers to low agreement or support of a particular experience as stated in the index label. Since all items were recoded in the same attitudinal direction, the means do not always correspond to the exact wording of the questionnaire items. Table 3.10 shows generally high correlations among items in each of the indexes concerning experiences in medical school. These high correlations are reflected in the substantial reliability coefficients reported in Table 3.11. This table of intercorrelations among measures concerning experiences in medical school indicates that each index correlates more highly with itself than with any other index or single-item measure, which is not surprising given the orthogonal factor solution.

Some single items that did not load highly on any factor or were not included in an index for theoretical reasons have been considered separately as single-item measures of school experiences. These include the following two items ranging in value from one to five: disagree with faculty—"I have been in agreement with medical school faculty and attending physicians on political issues concerning the profession of medicine" (never = high, with a mean and standard deviation of 2.89 and 0.62, respectively); and good grades in school—"What is your realistic appraisal of how well you have done overall in your course work compared to other members of your class?" (considerably better than average = high with a mean and standard deviation of 3.82 and 0.95, respectively).

Tangentially related to experiences in medical school are four other measures, not previously described, that have been included in the analysis and are aimed at explaining changes over time. These are debts expected upon completion of medical training (given in thousands with a mean of 10.43 and a standard deviation of 10.91); planning an academic research career (ranging in value from one to four with a

TABLE 3.10

Means and Standard Deviations for Indexes and for Items in Measures concerning Experiences in Medical School, with Inter-Item Correlations for Each Index, in Senior Year

Index and Item	Mean	Standard Deviation	Range of Value	Inter-Item Correlation, Item Number					
				2	3	4	5	6	7
Student treated badly by faculty	2.67	0.65	1-5						
1. As a medical student I have been treated as a mature and responsible adult by the faculty and attending physicians (never = high)	2.46	0.75	1-5	.65	.48	.38			
2. I have been pleased by the way the teaching faculty have treated me (never = high)	2.49	0.72	1-5	—	.50	.44			
3. My experience with the medical faculty and housestaff has been very supportive and encouraging (never = high)	2.49	0.71	1-5		—	.43			
4. To what extent have the teaching faculty and attending physicians been sensitive to you as a person as well as a medical student? (not at all = high)	2.62	0.69	1-4			—			
Patients treated badly by physicians	2.97	0.65	1-5						
1. I have been pleased with the way attending physicians have met the psychological and social needs of their patients (disagree = high)	3.50	1.16	1-5	.57	.34	.43			
2. Attending physicians have been good role models of how to interact with patients (never = high)	2.76	0.69	1-5	—	.38	.30			
3. During medical school, I have found myself getting angry at how patients were treated by physicians (always = high)	2.85	0.57	1-5		—	.24			
4. In treating patients at your school, to what extent are the psychological and social needs of the patient taken into account? (not at all = high)	2.35	0.67	1-4			—			
Student views career negatively	2.29	1.10	1-5						
1. Overall, I have greatly enjoyed my medical education (disagree = high)	2.19	1.24	1-5	.45					
2. I often have feelings or thoughts that I have chosen the wrong profession (agree = high)	2.39	1.35	1-5	—					
Experiencing difficulty in school	3.10	0.91	1-5						
1. Compared to your initial attitude upon entering medical school, do you now feel medical school has been overall: more, less, or about the same difficulty as you expected? (more = high)	1.90	0.77	1-3	.38	.19	.24	.32	.33	.29
2. How difficult was it for you to adjust to less free time for leisure and personal interests while in medical school? (extremely = high)	2.48	0.94	1-4	—	.28	.46	.64	.47	.49

	Mean	S.D.	Range	3	4	5	6	7
3. I feel I have sacrificed a great deal to become a physician (agree = high)	3.31	1.33	1-5	—	.30	.33	.27	.29
4. I have had enough free time during medical school to do the things I wanted (disagree = high)	3.16	1.30	1-5		—	.45	.42	.29

Please indicate how stressful each of the following has been for you since entering medical school:

	Mean	S.D.	Range	3	4	5	6	7
5. The shortage of time (stressful = high)	2.66	0.85	1-4			—	.58	.53
6. Balancing career and personal life (stressful = high)	2.79	0.87	1-4				—	.42
7. Working hard (stressful = high)	2.34	0.86	1-4					—

Support women's movement

	Mean	S.D.	Range	1	2
	2.69	0.83	1-4		
1. How familiar are you with the literature (like, Our Bodies, Ourselves) and issues of the women's health movement? (very = high)	2.35	1.05	1-4	—	.45
2. To what extent do you support the goals of the women's liberation movement? (a great deal = high)	3.03	0.90	1-4		—

Participate in liberal organizations

	Mean	S.D.	Range	1	2
	1.65	0.84	1-4		
1. During your medical training, to what extent have you participated in medical organizations or groups which have a politically liberal orientation (for example, Issues in Medicine, Student National Medical Association, American Women's Medical Association)? (a great deal = high)	1.61	0.89	1-4	—	.71
2. To what extent have you participated in formal organizations or informal groups (like support groups) which focus on issues affecting such minorities in medicine as women and blacks? (a great deal = high)	1.70	0.94	1-4		—

Ideological support from peers

Not all medical students have the same values upon entering medical school concerning the practice and profession of medicine. To what extent have each of the following groups supported and agreed with your initial ideas about the medical profession?

	Mean	S.D.	Range	1	2	3
	3.55	0.62	1-5			
1. Female classmates (agreed = high)	3.40	0.93	1-5	—	.21	.28
2. Male classmates (agreed = high)	3.37	0.87	1-5		—	.34
3. Your friends (agreed = high)	3.88	0.79	1-5			—

Note: All data are based on the responses of senior medical students who responded to both freshman and senior questionnaires. All data on items are calculated on approximately 279 cases (all those responding to both questionnaires minus nonrespondents). All data on indexes are based on exactly 279 cases, because nonrespondents are coded to the mean on each item. All items are coded in the same attitudinal direction as indicated in parentheses so that all correlations are positive and means are consistent with the index label.

In the case of items ranging from one to three or one to four included in indexes with values ranging from one to five, these items have been recoded in constructing indexes as follows. For items ranging from one to three, two was changed to three and three was changed to five. For items ranging from one to four, three was coded as four and four was coded as five. All correlations are significant at the .01 level.

TABLE 3.11

Intercorrelations of Measures concerning Experiences in Medical School in Senior Year

(reliabilities of indexes—Cronbach's alpha—reported on the diagonal of the matrix)

Variable	1	2	3	4	5	6	7	8	9
1. Student treated badly by faculty	(.79)	.53	.10	.37	.16	.14	-.00	.09	-.23
2. Patients treated badly by physicians		(.71)	.24	.16	.16	.12	-.06	.32	-.03
3. Student views career negatively			(.62)	.43	.17	.01	-.14	.16	-.37
4. Experiencing difficulty in school				(.81)	.20	.14	-.07	.13	-.32
5. Support women's movement					(.62)	.37	-.04	.25	-.04
6. Participated in liberal organizations						(.83)	.24	.15	-.10
7. Ideological support from peers							(.54)	-.16	.04
8. Disagree with faculty								(—)	-.14
9. Good grades in school									(—)

Note: All data are based on 279 cases, those who answered both freshman and senior questionnaires, except that data on "disagree with faculty" and "good grades in school" are calculated on 271 and 278 cases, respectively, because of nonresponses. These two variables are single-item measures; all others are indexes. All correlations of about .11 and higher are significant at the .05 probability level.

mean of 1.95 and a standard deviation of 0.87);* becoming more conservative in political outlook;[12] and perceiving faculty discouragement for primary-care medicine (ranging in value from one to five with a mean of 3.21 and a standard deviation of 1.03).†

SUMMARY

This chapter has outlined the data collection techniques and the measurement of all variables analyzed in this study. Questionnaire data for this longitudinal study were obtained from the vast majority of freshman medical students in the state of North Carolina in 1975 and again from these same students during their senior year. These two questionnaires were the culmination of numerous pretests and interviews with medical students, which aided in devising reliable measures.

The measurement description in this chapter has been detailed and rather lengthy because the author has developed new measures of professional orientations and medical school experiences. Most measures, although newly devised, have been shown to be very reliable. The data provide strong empirical support for the theoretical conception of professional values and expectations presented in Chapter 1.

Having completed the discussion of data collection and measurement, the author will present the study findings in the upcoming chapters. To begin, a description of the social backgrounds of the students and some differences between the schools are presented.

NOTES

1. Robert F. Winch and Donald T. Campbell, "Proof? No. Evidence? Yes. The Significance of Tests of Significance," The American Sociologist 4 (1969): 140-43.

2. Principal-factor solution with varimax rotation and iteration was used, producing a linear combination of variables that maximizes explained variance but does not assume that all the variance in any

---

*Planning an academic research career is an index composed of four items on the questionnaire given to seniors: questions 21(10) and 23(2, 10, 11). These items are highly intercorrelated with a reliability coefficient of .89.

†Discouragement for primary care is a two-item index composed of questions 46(1 and 2) on the senior questionnaire. These items are highly intercorrelated with a reliability coefficient of .88.

one variable is explained by the other variables in the matrix. There are numerous factoring techniques; however, principal-factor solution with iteration was chosen because it has a long history of use and is the most universally accepted factoring method. Norman Nie, C. Hadlai Hull, Jean Jenkins, Karin Steinbrenner, and Dale Bent, Statistical Package for the Social Sciences (New York: McGraw Hill, 1975), pp. 468-514. Furthermore, the results of the factor analysis were similar no matter which technique was chosen.

3. An eigenvalue is a measure of the relative importance of a factor in terms of how much of the total variance in the matrix it explains. An eigenvalue of at least one is a commonly accepted cut-off point for treating a factor as significant, since this ensures that only components explaining at least the total variance of one variable will be considered. Ibid., pp. 477-80.

4. For further details on the factor analysis, such as the factor loadings on each variable, see the author's dissertation, "Boys and Girls in White: Professional Orientation of the Student Physician" (Duke University, 1976).

5. For the calculation and a discussion of Cronbach's alpha, see David J. Armor, "Theta Reliability and Factor Scaling," in Sociological Methodology 1973-1974, ed. Herbert Costner (San Francisco: Jossey-Bass, 1974), pp. 17-26.

6. For a discussion of discriminant and convergent validation, see Donald T. Campbell and Donald W. Fiske, "Convergent and Discriminant Validation by the Mutlitrait-Multimethod Matrix," Psychological Bulletin 56 (1959): 81-105.

7. The socioeconomic index scores were based on the Duncan Scale. See Otis D. Duncan, "A Socioeconomic Index for All Occupations," in Occupations and Social Status, ed. Albert J. Reiss (New York: Free Press of Glencoe, 1961), pp. 109-38.

8. Douglas N. Jackson, Personality Research Form Manual (Goshen, N.Y.: Research Psychologists Press, 1974).

9. For a discussion of the Spearman-Brown prophecy formula, see Jum C. Nunnally, Psychometric Theory (New York: McGraw-Hill, 1967), pp. 172-205.

10. The cyncism scale was obtained from Edgar F. Borgatta and G. W. Bohrnstedt, unpublished manuscript (Madison, Wis.: Social Behavior Research Center, 1968).

11. A previous report indicates that this cyncism scale has a reliability of .67. Ibid.

12. Becoming more conservative on political outlook is a residualized change score, that is, political outlook at time two is regressed on political outlook at time one. Change in political outlook equals political outlook at time two - (a + [b * political outlook at time one]); where a is the intercept and b is the unstandardized regression coef-

ficient. A high score on this variable indicates becoming more conservative over time. For a discussion of residualized change scores,
see Lee J. Cronbach and Lita Furby, "How We Should Measure
'Change'—Or Should We?" Psychological Bulletin 74 (1970): 68–80.

4

ARRIVING STUDENTS:
WHO ARE THEY AND HOW DO THOSE
AT DIFFERENT SCHOOLS COMPARE?

As a prelude to examining the professional values and expectations of medical students, this rather brief chapter presents information on the respondents' social backgrounds. In addition, some initial comparisons are made among the three medical school freshman classes in North Carolina showing how their students differ in background and professional orientation. The three medical institutions that are compared are Duke University, the University of North Carolina (UNC) and Bowman Gray School of Medicine.

THE MEDICAL MAJORITY

Table 4.1 shows the percentages on selected social background characteristics of freshman medical students in total and by school. Traditionally, medical students in the United States have been primarily male, white, Protestant, and from upper-class families. Since medical school admission committees have been publicly pressured to recruit some underrepresented groups like women and blacks, the medical students in North Carolina in 1975, like the medical students nationally, were somewhat less homogeneous than in previous years. National data on the freshman medical school classes in 1970 revealed that 11.1 percent were women and 6.1 percent were blacks. [1] Table 4.1 indicates that efforts five years later in North Carolina to recruit minorities have more successfully increased the proportion of women (25.8 percent) than that of blacks (8.9 percent). The percentage of women and blacks in the sample is similar to the 1975 nationwide first-year medical school female and black enrollment of 23.8 percent and 6.8 percent respectively. [2] Furthermore, we note that nationally, as well as in North Carolina, affirmative action has

TABLE 4.1

Percentages on Social Background Characteristics in Total and by School
for Freshman Medical Students, 1975

Social Background Characteristics	Duke	University of North Carolina	Bowman Gray	Total
Sex				
Male	68.5	78.0	75.0	74.2
Female	31.5	22.0	25.0	25.8
Race				
White	91.9	87.0	97.1	91.1
Black	8.1	13.0	2.9	8.9
Age				
23 or less	94.2	63.8	81.7[a]	78.0
24 or more	5.8	36.2	18.3	22.0
Marital status				
Single	84.1	67.8	73.6[b]	74.5
Married	15.9	32.2	26.4	25.5
Background				
Rural	8.1	15.2	15.3[b]	13.0
Small town	21.8	34.8	34.7	30.7
Medium-city suburb	13.8	4.2	8.3	8.3
Medium city	24.1	28.0	13.9	23.1
Large-city suburb	24.1	14.4	13.9	17.3
Large city	8.1	3.4	13.9	7.6
Religion				
Protestant	64.0	82.1	77.5[b]	75.1
Catholic	21.3	9.4	12.7	14.1
Jewish	11.2	7.7	5.6	8.3
None	3.4	0.9	4.2	2.5
Religiosity				
Important	52.8	62.7	73.2[a]	62.2
Not important	47.2	37.3	26.8	37.8
Father's education				
High school or less	7.9	31.4	31.9[a]	24.0
College (one to four years)	30.3	27.1	47.2	33.3
Postgraduate (one or more years)	61.8	41.5	20.8	42.7
Mother's education				
High school or less	16.9	30.5	36.1[a]	27.6
College (one to four years)	52.8	43.2	54.2	49.1
Postgraduate (one or more years)	30.3	26.3	9.7	23.3
Doctor in family				
Yes	43.8	33.9	34.7	37.3
No	56.2	66.1	65.3	62.7
Number[c]	89	118	72	279

[a] $p \leq .01$ of a significant difference between the schools from one-way analysis of variance.

[b] $p \leq .05$ of a significant difference between the schools from one-way analysis of variance.

[c] In some cases percentages are calculated on slightly fewer cases than those indicated here because of missing data.

worked better for women than for blacks. Other racial minority
groups, including American Indians and Asians, compose only 2.5
percent of the sample. The three medical schools do not differ significantly in their recruitment of minorities, although UNC recruits
a slightly greater percentage of blacks and Duke selects proportionally
more females.

Most students are 22 when they enter school; the rest range in
age from 20 to 32 years. Few students (22.0 percent) are over 24 at
the beginning of first year, although UNC selected the oldest freshman
class in 1975. Consistent with UNC's older cohort, freshmen at that
school were more likely to be married. The marital status of students
tends to parallel their age status at all schools, so that the younger
the student body the more single (never married) students there are.
Most students are, therefore, young and also single.

Many respondents are from rural areas or small towns of less
than 50,000 population (43.7 percent), owing somewhat to the numerous small towns and rural areas in close proximity to these medical
schools. Of the students from both UNC and Bowman Gray, 50 percent are from small towns and rural areas compared with only 30 percent at Duke. Duke selects more of their students from urban areas
outside North Carolina consistent with their prestigious national reputation and with their research and specialty-medicine focus. As a
state school, UNC receives proportionally more applications from
in-state students, many of whom are from rural areas. Although
Bowman Gray, like Duke, is a private school, it appears more committed than Duke to improving the underrepresentation of physicians
from small towns and rural locales. This is in part due to Bowman
Gray's less prestigious reputation, to their primary-care emphasis,
and to their greater state allotment for admitting North Carolina students.

Table 4.1 also shows that most medical students are Protestant
(75.1 percent), with a minority indicating they are Catholic (14.1 percent) or Jewish (8.3 percent). Duke enrolls proportionally more Catholic and Jewish students, probably a reflection of their more urban
student population. Furthermore, when asked to evaluate the importance of religion in their lives, most students (62.2 percent) indicate
at least some importance. Consistent with the rural and small-town
origins of those at UNC and Bowman Gray, these students tend to be
the most religious.

As expected, students are generally from highly educated and
professional families. Few students' fathers or mothers have had
no education beyond high school (24.0 percent and 27.6 percent respectively). Many fathers have had at least some postgraduate training beyond college (42.7 percent). When asked to indicate their father's occupation, 49 percent listed professional or technical careers

and 25 percent mentioned manager, official, or proprietor of a business. About half of the students' mothers are housewives. Of the mothers who work outside the home, 63 percent are in professional or technical careers. Compared with the other two schools, Duke students are from more highly educated families consistent with their more urban backgrounds. As a group, medical students are from the most privileged classes in society.

Finally, Table 4.1 indicates that many students (37.3 percent) report at least one physician relative in their family. Furthermore, 18 percent of all fathers and 6 percent of all working mothers are physicians. Physicians and other professionals appear to spawn new generations of doctors. The children of the working classes are less likely to achieve the privileged status of physician.

The educational and occupational backgrounds of all respondents' parents closely approximate national data on freshman medical students for the same year.[3] Since the respondents in this study appear similar in their socioeconomic and minority statuses to nationwide first-year medical school classes, we can have more confidence in the representativeness of the North Carolina sample.

SCHOOL DIFFERENCES ON FRESHMEN'S PROFESSIONAL ORIENTATIONS

Since the freshman questionnaires were administered during the first week of school, initial professional orientation differences among the three medical institutions' classes cannot be attributed to variations in professional socialization. For the most part, freshman orientation differences between the schools do not persist when controlling on social background variables. In other words, variations among institutions on their freshmen's professional orientations are primarily a function of students' differing backgrounds. School differences on professional orientations that cannot be accounted for by variations in students' social backgrounds reflect differential self-selection and school selection policies.

After controlling for social background attributes, initial school differences are significant on only two of the professional orientations examined in this study. These are expectations to practice primary-care medicine and the belief that patients should not have absolute confidence in physicians' judgments. Duke students begin school less oriented to primary-care medicine (as indicated by their mean primary-care score of 3.39 on a one-to-five scale) than students at UNC (4.06) and Bowman Gray (4.10). This finding is not surprising because Duke selects students more oriented to academic medicine and research because of its combined medical and doctoral degree program. Thus self-selection and school selection policies account for this differential interest in primary-care medicine at the onset of training. In Chapter 6, we shall see that during training Duke students find faculty and housestaff less encouraging of primary-care medicine than students at the other two schools. Thus, the message to students upon entrance to school and later during training is that Duke is primarily concerned with training researchers and specialists.

Differences on social background attributes also do not explain why Duke students begin school more critical of patients having absolute confidence in physicians' judgments (the mean for Duke on this index ranging from one to five is 3.19, compared with the UNC mean of 2.74 and the Bowman Gray mean of 2.48). For some reason not obvious to the author, the Duke admissions committee appears to—consciously or unconsciously—select students who are more critical about physicians' judgments than do the other admissions boards.

SUMMARY

To summarize, the typical freshman medical student in this study is male, white, 22 years old, single, from a small to medium city, Protestant, somewhat religious, and from an upperclass family. Due to affirmative action programs and to the greater number of minority medical applications, blacks and especially women are increasingly represented in medical school classes.

Compared to the other two schools, Duke attracts students who are more likely to be young, unmarried, and from upperclass families and less likely to be from rural or small-town areas, Protestant, or religious. Generally students at UNC and Bowman Gray vary little from each other on these background attributes. On the average, UNC students are substantially older and somewhat more likely to be married than students at the other schools. Differential selection policies and self-selection account for the social background differences among the three medical schools. By and large, professional orientation differences between the schools are accounted for by variations on social background attributes, although Duke students begin less interested in primary-care medicine.

NOTES

1. W. F. Dubé, "U.S. Medical Student Enrollment, 1970-71 through 1974-75 (Datagram)," Journal of Medical Education 50 (1975): 303-06.

2. Travis L. Gordon and W. F. Dubé, "Medical Student Enrollment, 1971-72 through 1975-76 (Datagram)," Journal of Medical Education 51 (1976): 144-46.

3. W. F. Dubé, Descriptive Study of Enrolled Medical Students 1975-6 (Washington, D. C.: Association of American Medical Colleges, 1977), pp. 57-62.

5

ENTERING AND LEAVING
MEDICAL SCHOOL: CHANGES IN
PROFESSIONAL ORIENTATIONS

Do students begin medical school with a somewhat liberal and idealistic orientation to practice and professional issues? Do they become more conservative and less concerned with the needs of patients during their four years of training? The answers to these questions are, to a large extent, yes, depending on the particular professional values and expectations considered. In this chapter, students' professional orientations upon entrance to and graduation from medical school are described in order to assess the effects of professional socialization. The findings will help shed light on the conflicting views of socialization presented in previous research, that is, the image of medical education as an orderly process whereby students acquire dominant professional ideologies versus the problematic view that medical training does not produce major and lasting attitudinal shifts. In addition to determining which values and expectations change during medical school, the author will focus on what implications for health care, medical education, and the profession can be drawn from these findings.

The presentation of findings will be organized by health-care problem areas, that is, physicians' relationships with patients, political and economic issues, sexism in medicine, and physician maldistribution. The three medical schools are combined in the data analysis since school variations over time are discussed in Chapter 6 with an analysis showing why shifts in orientation occur.

Tables 5.1 to 5.4 present the means, standard deviations, and percentage distributions for all respondents on professional orientation measures during both their freshman and senior years, the correlation of each measure from time one to time two, and the T-test for dependent samples indicating significant differences in the means over time. The T-tests show whether the group as a whole changes on a particular orientation from freshman to senior year. This is a problematic measure of change because it is possible for the group means to be the same during both years when in fact many individuals have fluctuated in their opinions. Thus, if all those who scored high on a particular variable at time one scored low at time two and vice versa, substantial individual change would be masked by identical means across time. To remedy this situation, correlation coefficients for each measure across time have been computed. The correlations indicate to what extent individuals have scored the same on variables from freshman to senior year so that a high correlation indicates little individual fluctuation. With these two measures, it can be determined if change occurs because the whole group changes uniformly (significant T-test, high correlation), individuals fluctuate over time but the group as a whole remains the same (T-test nonsignificant, low correlation), or both individual and group change is evidenced (significant T-test, low correlation).

PHYSICIANS' RELATIONSHIPS WITH PATIENTS

Medical schools have been criticized for their lack of attention to the problems of humanizing and equalizing doctor/patient interactions, that is, treating the patient as a person and not a disease entity. Providing patients with more health information, advocating a more critical appraisal of physicians, paying attention to patients' social and psychological problems, and wanting to help others are values that may help humanize and equalize physicians' relationships with patients.

Consistent with previous research,[1] Table 5.1 shows that almost all students had begun medical school espousing humanistic values. Almost all (over 90 percent) placed importance on helping people and on social and psychological factors in health care, including the value of rapport and empathy with patients. This finding is not surprising because idealistic humanism is the socially accepted response due to the subtle pressure on medical professionals to at least espouse concern for the human side of patient care.

From freshman to senior year, little change is evident on these humanistic patient-care values. Seniors viewed helping people as somewhat less focal to their careers than originally, although most still expressed this ideal upon completion of school (80.3 percent). Like their earlier responses, almost all seniors emphasized the importance of social and psychological factors in treating patients. When students were asked whether physicians at their school have been good role models in terms of paying attention to patients' social and psychological needs, relatively few students (33 percent) responded

TABLE 5.1

Means, Standard Deviations, and Percentage Distributions on Measures concerning the Doctor/Patient Relationship during Medical Students' Freshman and Senior Years, 1975 and 1978 (with correlation coefficients between measures across time and T-test for dependent samples)

| | Freshman Year 1975 | | | | | Senior Year 1978 | | | | | | |
| | Index Score[a] | | Percentage in Each Category | | | Index Score | | Percentage in Each Category | | | | |
Variable	Mean	Standard Deviation	Disagree	Neutral	Agree	Mean	Standard Deviation	Disagree	Neutral	Agree	T-Test	r
Important to provide health information to patients	3.27	0.79	22.6	36.2	41.2	3.30	0.78	20.8	28.7	50.5	0.55	.42
Patients should not have absolute confidence in physicians' judgments	2.82	1.08	46.2	19.0	34.8	3.36	1.01	25.8	22.9	51.3	8.15[b]	.43
Social and psychological factors, including empathy, are important in health care	4.32	0.55	—	7.9	92.1	4.33	0.58	0.4	9.7	90.0	0.11	.37
Chose medicine in order to help people (helping people is important part of medical career)[c]	3.34	0.58	9.3	—[a]	90.7	3.13	0.63	19.7	—	80.3	5.55[b]	.43

r = correlation coefficient

[a] All variables are indexes composed of two or more questionnaire items calculated on 279 cases. The range of possible values is one to five for all measures except choosing medicine in order to help people, which ranges from one to four. On indexes ranging from one to five, scores of 1.0 to 2.50 are labeled "disagree"; scores of 2.51 to 3.49 are labeled "neutral"; and scores of 3.50 to 5.0 are labeled "agree." On the measure coded from one to four, scores of 1.0 to 2.50 are labeled "disagree," and scores of 2.51 to 4.0 are labeled "agree."

[b] $p < .001$.

[c] Approximate wording on 1975 questionnaire shown with approximate wording on 1978 questionnaire in parentheses.

affirmatively. * Consistent with a problematic view of socialization, students retained their initial humanistic ideals despite negative role models. The medium-level correlations on values of humanizing doctor/patient relationships are more likely due to the low variance on these indexes than to individual fluctuation.

One assumption of this research is that informing patients about their health and not expecting their absolute confidence would reduce the knowledge and authority distinctions between physicians and patients as well as involve patients in their own treatment and in preventive medical action. Table 5.1 indicates that first-year students have tended to place importance on providing health information concerning diagnosis and treatment to patients, including giving patients access to their medical records (41.2 percent). On the other hand, the same students tended to advocate absolute patient confidence in physicians' judgments, including the taboo on criticizing colleagues in public (46.2 percent).

Although individuals have fluctuated somewhat in their views toward providing health information to patients, † little overall group change is evident on this variable from freshman to senior year. Whereas some students have become more adamant about a patient's rights to be told everything, other students have begun to feel that exceptions to this rule are appropriate.

On the issue of patient confidence in physicians' judgments, however, seniors were much more critical of absolute confidence in physicians (51.3 percent) than they were as freshmen (34.8 percent). These sentiments were echoed in the interviews with senior medical students. When asked how and why their values have changed since freshman year, most students said they were less naive and more realistic about the limitations of medical practice and more aware of medical malpractice. The greater realism among students was reflected in the following two comments made by a female and a male medical student, respectively.

> I seem to have a more realistic picture of what medicine
> is like than I had before . . . so I guess my attitudes may

---

*This measure concerning physicians' treatment of patients is described in Chapter 3. It is a four-item index that has been divided into categories low, neutral, and high. "Thirty-three percent" refers to those scoring low on perceiving faculty as negative role models.

† The somewhat low correlations over time on both measures involving the equalization of doctor/patient relationships may indicate measurement error more than individual fluctuation because both measures have somewhat low reliabilities freshman and senior years. (The alphas range from .52 to .60 as shown in Chapter 3.)

have changed somewhat. I had some general ideas that
medicine was something good, that it was going to help a
lot of people . . . that it would have a lot of answers to a
lot of problems. And then I think I was struck by the fact
that a lot of medicine here is diagnostic and not so much
therapeutic. . . . We spend so much time and effort and
money finding out what does the patient have and giving
him a diagnosis and then a lot of times you can't offer them
much. You can't really give them a cure.

My initial impression of the way medicine was practiced
does not coincide with what I've found to be fact in the last
four years here. I think everyone is sort of idealistic
about the practice of medicine and I've lost a lot of that
idealism since I've been in medical school. It's just not
everything it's cracked up to be. It used to be sort of a
mystique, an unknown. . . . But now after being in it
for several years, it's really not that at all. I've found
that doctors are just as much human beings as other people are. . . . My clinical exposure has really had a great
deal to do with my impression right now of what medicine
is . . . seeing how medicine is practiced or not practiced in certain areas.

Seniors seeming more aware of the limitations of medical
practice might account for their becoming more tolerant of patient
skepticism about physicians' judgments. Fears of medical malpractice may also lead students to want less absolute reliance on
their judgments. In any case, involving patients in health care by
giving them health information and by supporting less than total confidence in physicians should help equalize the doctor/patient relationship, if students put their beliefs into practice.

Using a variety of measures, some authors have found that
medical students become more cynical and less benevolent as they go
through training, regardless of whether the authors consider this a
temporary adjustment to medical school.[2] Students in the present
study have become much more realistic about the limits of medical
practice, as indicated by their greater acceptance of criticism toward
physicians, but only slightly less idealistic in their career goals to
help people. Likewise, students scored slightly more cynically over
time on a personality measure (the belief that most people try to use
others to get ahead), although most seniors still ranked rather low
on cynicism.* Thus, students maintained most of their humanistic

---

*The personality measure of cynicism is an index ranging from
one to four with a freshman and senior mean of 1.60 and 1.76, respectively. There is little variation on this measure in both years

idealism but at the same time became more realistic about the limits of physicians' expertise. It appears that the idealism/cynicism continuum is a more complex construct than previous studies have indicated. Researchers need to clearly define the labels cyncism, realism, and idealism before making broad generalizations about the effects of the socialization process on these orientations.

In summary, senior students overall showed the same degree of interest in providing health information to patients and in dealing with the social and psychological factors in health care that they did at beginning medical school. Even though medical educators have been criticized for not emphasizing ways to communicate with patients, and few students report that their mentors have been good role models when it came to dealing with the social and psychological dynamics in illness, this appeared to have little overall effect on students' values. Thus, professional socialization did not seem to adversely affect students with respect to their humanitarian and egalitarian values of patient care.

Because most seniors recognized the importance of giving health information to patients concerning diagnosis and treatment, of understanding patients' social and psychological problems, and of patients being critical of their physicians, we might expect that in future practice these students will be more humanistic and egalitarian in interacting with patients. But if students are not provided good role models in terms of the interpersonal aspects of patient care, one wonders if students will be able to put their ideals into practice. Furthermore, the rigorous nature of postmedical training, where often there is little time for doctor/patient interactions, may undermine these students' best intentions. Whether students can maintain these egalitarian and humanistic orientations and implement them in practice remains to be seen.

Although seniors viewed helping people as somewhat less focal to their careers than originally, most students still expressed this ideal during their senior year. The extent to which this idealistic desire to help people translates into supporting social reforms in medicine and making personal sacrifices for the public good is discussed next.

POLITICAL AND ECONOMIC CHANGE IN THE MEDICAL PROFESSION

Controversial reforms concerning government intervention in medicine, changing the profit organization of health services, and

---

as indicated by the standard deviations for freshman (.42) and senior years (.47).

TABLE 5.2

Means, Standard Deviations, and Percentage Distributions on Measures concerning Political and Economic Change in the Medical Profession during Medical Students' Freshman and Senior Years, 1975 and 1978

(with correlation coefficients between measures across time and T-test for dependent samples)

| | Freshman Year 1975 | | | | | Senior Year 1978 | | | | | | |
| | Index Score[a] | | Percentage in Each Category | | | Index Score | | Percentage in Each Category | | | | |
Variable	Mean	Standard Deviation	Low	Middle	High	Mean	Standard Deviation	Low	Middle	High	T-Test	r
Profession's control over health services should be reduced through government intervention and socialized medicine	2.96	1.03	35.1	31.9	33.0	2.54	1.00	52.3	25.4	22.2	7.84[b]	.60
Favor a compulsory National Service Corps for physicians to serve in deprived areas	1.95	0.66	24.7	55.6	19.6	1.72	0.72	43.3	40.8	15.9	4.73[b]	.37
The health-care system needs to be changed so that profits cannot be made	2.98	1.24	45.7	13.3	41.0	2.40	1.17	66.3	10.8	22.9	8.22[b]	.53
Physicians' status and financial rewards need to be lowered	3.08	0.82	30.8	32.3	36.9	2.76	0.85	44.1	31.9	24.0	7.35[b]	.63
High status and income were important in career selection (high status and income are important part of medical career)[c]	1.94	0.59	77.8	—	22.2	2.12	0.59	70.3	—	29.7	5.38[b]	.57
Expect to work for political and social change in medicine	2.17	0.74	68.8	—	31.2	1.86	0.73	81.0	—	19.0	7.58[b]	.57
Percentage of time expect to do volunteer work	17.51	11.55	38.6	37.5	23.9	11.40	7.93	67.6	24.6	7.7	9.51[b]	.48

r = correlation coefficient

[a]Variables are indexes composed of two or more questionnaire items with the exception of favoring a National Service Corps, favoring a change in the health-care system, and planning volunteer work, which are single-item measures. All calculations are based on 279 cases, with the exception of the single items that are computed on slightly fewer cases because of missing data. The range of possible values is one to five on favoring government intervention, a change in the health-care system, and lower financial rewards for physicians. On these measures, scores of 1.0 to 2.50 are labeled "low"; scores of 2.51 to 3.49 are labeled "middle"; and scores of 3.50 to 5.0 are labeled "high." The range of possible values is one to four on the importance of high status and income and expecting to work for change. On these measures, scores of 1.0 to 2.50 are labeled "low," and scores of 2.51 to 4.0 are labeled "high." The single item favoring a National Service Corps ranges from one to three so that the three responses "no," "yes, only if medical education is paid," and "yes," are labeled "low," "middle," and "high," respectively. The percentage of time one plans volunteer work has a possible range from 0 to 100 percent so that 0 to 10 percent is labeled "low"; 11 to 20 percent is labeled "middle"; and 21 percent and over is labeled "high."

[b]p < .001.

[c]Approximate wording on 1975 questionnaire shown with approximate wording on 1978 questionnaire in parentheses.

92

lowering physicians' incomes and status address major problems with the current health-care system. Critics advocate changing these political and economic features of the health-care system in order to aid such problems as physician maldistribution, the quality of medical care, and rising medical costs. Some solutions to the current crisis in health care also call for the selection of medical students with less personal interest in money and status and with greater commitment to provide voluntary medical services and to work for political and social change in medicine.

As indicated in Table 5.2, the medical schools in the present study seem to have selected students with somewhat liberal orientations on issues concerning political and economic change in medicine. The freshman medical students were fairly evenly divided on most change issues so that 33 percent, 41 percent, and 37 percent, respectively, favored government intervention to reduce the profession's control over health services; change in the health-care system so that drug companies, insurance companies, and hospitals could not make profits; and lowering physicians' status and financial rewards. Furthermore, most first-year students (55.6 percent) advocated a National Service Corps that would have required all physicians to serve one or two years in a medically deprived area if medical education was paid for by the government. Few (19.6 percent) favored such a plan without remuneration. These findings support those in previous research that show about half the entering medical students are liberal on issues of political and economic change in medicine.[3]

Also consistent with previous studies,[4] few freshman medical students (22.2 percent) admitted to choosing medicine for the status and financial rewards. This finding is not surprising because it is socially taboo for medical students to express interest in pecuniary achievements. Physicians are supposed to be motivated by higher goals, such as helping mankind or intellectual challenge, although they have been criticized by many for their interests in wealth rather than health. Medical students' stated reasons for choosing medicine are thus consistent with approved social values.

Although most freshmen denied personal monetary and status motivations (77.8 percent), far fewer advocated the lowering of physicians' high status and incomes (36.9 percent). Students may not have selected medicine for financial reasons, but most did not oppose this fringe benefit. Contrasting students' personal economic motivations for choosing medicine with their attitudes about the amount of money and prestige deserved by physicians has revealed a more realistic portrayal of medical students than has previous research. Medical students have been described in other studies as extremely benevolent and uninterested in money. In choosing to delve deeper into students' economic orientations, the author has challenged the functionalists' acceptance of medical altruism (see Chapter 1 for a discussion of functionalism).

Contrary to expectation, students appeared almost as likely to plan to work for political and social change in medicine as to advocate liberal changes. In freshman year, 31 percent of the students were at least somewhat interested in working for political and social change. In addition, the average percentage of practice time that freshmen planned to do volunteer work as physicians, that is, working in free clinics and giving free care to the needy, was a high 17.5 percent. Translated into hours, in a 60-hour week (the average amount of time that freshmen expected to work after medical training) freshmen planned to work 10.5 hours for free. These plans are consistent with students' initial humanitarianism and liberalism upon entrance to medical school.

From freshman to senior year, students as a whole became substantially more conservative on all values and expectations concerning political and economic change in medicine, as indicated by the change in means and the high correlations between time 1 and time 2 measures.* Whereas one-third to two-fifths of the freshmen initially favored a reduction in the profession's control over health care, a change in the profit system, and lower physician status and financial rewards, less than one-fourth of the seniors favored these reforms. In addition, only 25 percent of the freshmen were opposed to a National Service Corps for physicians, but by senior year 43 percent were opposed to this plan. These findings are consistent with previous longitudinal data showing greater student conservatism in the senior year on issues of government intervention in health care.[5]

As a prior study,[6] seniors were only a little more likely to acknowledge the importance of financial considerations in their medical careers (29.7 percent) than they were as freshmen (22.2 percent). Although the vast majority of seniors were still reticent to express these personal financial concerns, few would agree to lower physicians' incomes and status (24.0 percent). Thus, seniors might not admit that they consider financial rewards important, but they do expect and advocate the large economic advantages that physicians accrue.

Students also became more conservative in their career plans as they went through medical training. Whereas 31 percent of the

---

*The single-item measures have slightly lower correlations over time than the indexes. This is partially an artifact of measurement error due to the lower reliability of single-item measures rather than an indication of greater individual fluctuation over time.

students began school expecting to work for political and social change, only 19 percent planned political work by the senior year. Likewise, the percentage of time students expected to do volunteer work decreased dramatically over time so that seniors planned an average of only 11.4 percent of their practice time for volunteer service compared with 17.5 percent when they entered school. Thus, for a 60-hour work week, seniors planned to spend only 6.8 hours in volunteer service compared with 10.5 hours originally.

Most seniors espoused altruistic values, but when they were questioned about their practice plans, the notion of the altruistic medical student wore a little thin. Students became only slightly less committed to humanitarian service (helping people), but their interests waned more dramatically on specific plans to help people through volunteer and political work. As shown later, their interests declined on practices in need areas also. General humanitarian values, therefore, do not necessarily reflect much social concern, since students have become less likely to support or see themselves working for reforms of the medical profession aimed at helping the poor. A distinction needs to be made between wanting to help individual clients as some vague ideal and realistically planning a socially committed practice to meet public needs.

During interviews, senior medical students were asked if they thought most medical students at their school had become more or less conservative on practice and professional issues since entering school. Consistent with the survey findings already reported, the overwhelming majority said students had become more conservative. Many mentioned the conservative nature of medical school, the profession, and the role models as strong socializing influences. The following comments made during separate interviews with two males and one female, respectively, illustrate the conservative nature of professional socialization in medical school.

> In many ways you are programmed to fit into a mold here and that mold is a lot more conservative than the ideas that people come in here with. . . . Pressure comes in part from the senior staff and in part . . . from the big medical-center mold. There is a push toward research; there is a push toward shuffling patients in and shuffling patients out as fast as possible and still maintaining their health care.

> I think that most people that go through the rigor of four years of medical school tend to become more conservative. . . . Doctors as professional people are very conservative at least on an outward appearance. . . . It's

hard to be a liberal or radical when you're locked in with a group of conservatives. Being around people of that nature for about four years, you tend to take on a lot of their characteristics without ever realizing that in fact you have incorporated many of these same feelings and ideas.

I guess there is a general trend toward conservatism. Even the people who are more liberal . . . I think that they have had to change their appearances somewhat, change their conduct somewhat to conform to the medical role. . . . I think that just being around here in this conservative environment helps solidify people toward the more conservative aspect. . . . I sort of get the impression that it is a very conservative field, which I didn't realize before.

Thus, the image of medicine and medical school as conservative institutions was a recurring theme. In fact, few seniors in this study rated the political atmosphere of their school as liberal (15.0 percent); most indicated either middle of the road (53.6 percent) or conservative (31.4 percent). * Thus, it is not surprising that students have become more conservative in their values and expectations concerning political and economic change in the profession of medicine. These findings support the view of socialization as an orderly process whereby dominant values are acquired; students on the whole have come closer to adopting traditional professional views, that is, political and economic status quo in the organization of medicine. As physicians in practice, most of these students are not likely to push for radical or even liberal changes in the profession. Furthermore, medical education seems to have a detrimental effect on students' social service plans.

It is worthwhile noting that although most of the students interviewed felt that others had become more conservative, few admitted that they had also succumbed to such changes. Medical students may not want to admit to becoming more conservative if they view it as a sign of aging or as a sign of losing their ideals. The previous political era of the late 1960s and early 1970s has made being liberal the more socially acceptable stance for many who grew up during that time. Since medical students seem somewhat reluctant to admit growing conservatism, studies that ask students or physicians to rate

---

*The number of students responding to this item was 274. The item states, "Overall, is the political atmosphere at your school: (1) liberal, (2) middle of the road, (3) conservative."

their change in political orientation over time cannot substitute for a longitudinal approach.

PREJUDICE AGAINST WOMEN
PHYSICIANS AND PATIENTS

The medical profession has been criticized for its prejudicial treatment of women physicians and patients. The increasing number of female physicians and the women's liberation movement have generally increased sensitivity to such issues as the pressure on women to choose traditionally "female" specialties (such as pediatrics), the need for more women doctors, and gynecologists' patronizing treatment of patients including their inaccurate view of female sexuality.

Table 5.3 shows that although the vast majority of freshmen (79.2 percent) agreed that more women doctors are needed, they were less likely to acknowledge that women physicians or patients experience prejudicial treatment. Thus, only 39 percent concurred that medicine is harder for women due to professional and public prejudice against women physicians. About 43 percent agreed that women experience pressure to choose pediatrics and pressure not to choose surgery. Finally, only 29 percent acknowledged that physicians often treat their women patients in a patronizing way. Although freshmen were fairly evenly divided on the general issue of medicine being harder for women due to prejudice against women physicians, comparing items in this index shows that they were more likely to acknowledge patient bias (54.5 percent) as opposed to professional bias (35.7 percent). *

The most striking feature about the freshmen responses to the items in the indexes concerning specialty choice pressure on women physicians and discrimination against women patients is the large proportion of students expressing no opinion—ranging from 25.5 percent to 48.7 percent. † The large neutral-opinion response on these issues indicates that many students were probably unaware of these discrimination problems upon entrance to school. Most students, however, have recognized the need for more women doctors.

---

*The items in the index concerning professional and public prejudice against women physicians range from one to five on an agree-to-disagree scale that includes a neutral category. The percentages reported here refer to all those agreeing somewhat or strongly to these items.

† Table 7.4 shows the percentage distribution broken down by sex in categories "agree," "neutral," and "disagree" on items in these women's indexes.

TABLE 5.3

Means, Standard Deviations, and Percentage Distributions on Measures concerning the Treatment of Women Physicians and Patients during Medical Students' Freshman and Senior Years, 1975 and 1978 (with correlation coefficients between measures across time and T-test for dependent samples)

	Freshman Year 1975					Senior Year 1978					T-Test	r
	Index Score[a]		Percentage in Each Category			Index Score		Percentage in Each Category				
Variable	Mean	Standard Deviation	Disagree	Neutral	Agree	Mean	Standard Deviation	Disagree	Neutral	Agree		
There is professional and public prejudice against women physicians	3.00	.91	35.5	25.4	39.1	2.92	1.04	41.2	21.9	36.9	1.11	.26
There is pressure on women physicians to choose certain fields, such as pediatrics	3.20	.89	23.3	34.1	42.7	3.16	1.16	33.3	20.1	46.6	0.56	.30
There is a need for more women physicians in this country	4.00	.92	10.8	10.0	79.2	3.79	1.02	15.4	15.1	69.5	4.14[b]	.64
Physicians generally treat women patients in a patronizing and prejudicial way	3.04	.71	28.3	42.7	29.0	3.11	0.95	34.4	27.6	38.0	1.46	.49

r = correlation coefficient

[a] All variables are indexes composed of two or more questionnaire items calculated on 279 cases. The range of possible values is one to five for all measures. Scores of 1.0 to 2.50 are labeled "disagree"; scores of 2.51 to 3.49 are labeled "neutral"; and scores of 3.50 to 5.0 are labeled "agree."

[b] p < .001.

Contrary to the author's expectations, students as a group have not become more sensitive to issues of sex discrimination over time. In fact, students overall did not change their views on these issues except that seniors were somewhat less in favor of increasing the number of women physicians (69.5 percent) than they were as freshmen (79.2 percent). The generally low correlations between freshman- and senior-year measures concerning discrimination toward women doctors, however, indicated some individual and subgroup fluctuation masked by the stability of the group means. Thus, some students have found conditions for women physicians better than they expected and some have found things worse. In Chapter 7, the author will explore how particular groups, such as women, tend to fluctuate differently than men on issues of sexism in medicine.

Although a large proportion of the freshmen had no opinion on items concerning specialty pressure and discrimination against women patients (ranging from 25.5 percent to 48.7 percent), few seniors responded with a neutral view on these issues (ranging from 7.6 percent to 26.1 percent). Interviews conducted with medical students suggested that the presence of women in medical school has contributed to sensitizing students about women's issues, even if not always in a sympathetic way. Seeing or not seeing evidence of discrimination toward women has contributed to students' perceptions that conditions were worse or better than they had expected. The recently improved conditions for women at some medical schools, including less overt discrimination, may also account for some seniors' decreased concern with these women's issues. In fact, only 23 percent of the seniors felt that teaching faculty and attending physicians had been a little or moderately racist or sexist. * Thus, medical students as a whole are not likely to be instrumental in alleviating sexism in medicine because as a group they are not overly concerned about women's problems.

PHYSICIAN MALDISTRIBUTION

Since the shortages of physicians in primary-care medicine and in rural and inner-city ghetto areas are critical health problems in the United States today, medical students' practice plans have definite

---

*There were 278 students who responded to this discrimination item, which asks, "To what extent have the teaching faculty and attending physicians been racist or sexist?" The responses on a four-point scale included "not at all," "a little," "a moderate amount," and "a great deal."

TABLE 5.4

Means, Standard Deviations, and Percentage Distributions on Measures concerning Physician Maldistribution during Medical Students' Freshman and Senior Years, 1975 and 1978

(with correlation coefficients between measures across time and T-test for dependent samples)

Variable	Freshman Year 1975					Senior Year 1978						
	Index Score[a]		Percentage in Each Category			Index Score		Percentage in Each Category				
	Mean	Standard Deviation	Disagree	Neutral	Agree	Mean	Standard Deviation	Disagree	Neutral	Agree	T-Test	r
Expect to practice primary-care medicine	3.86	1.13	18.6	8.6	72.8	3.25	1.52	40.5	8.6	50.9	6.87[b]	.41
Expect a rural practice	2.56	1.00	45.5	—	54.5	2.06	1.02	65.8	—	34.2	8.01[b]	.49
Expect an inner-city ghetto practice	1.96	0.79	75.9	—	24.1	1.53	0.80	84.9	—	15.1	8.78[b]	.47
Committed to choosing a specialty and geographic area that need physicians	3.61	1.05	21.1	17.9	60.9	3.11	1.25	39.1	19.7	41.2	7.45[b]	.55

r = correlation coefficient

[a] Variables are indexes composed of two or more questionnaire items, with the exception of rural-practice and inner-city ghetto-practice expectations, which are single-item measures. Calculations are based on 279 cases, with the exception of rural-practice and inner-city ghetto-practice expectations, which are computed on 278 cases. The range of possible values is one to five for all measures, except for the single-item variables, which range from one to four. On indexes ranging from one to five, scores of 1.0 to 2.50 are labeled "disagree"; scores of 2.51 to 3.49 are labeled "neutral"; and scores of 3.50 to 5.0 are labeled "agree." On measures coded from one to four, responses of very unlikely and somewhat unlikely are labeled "disagree" and responses of very likely and somewhat likely are labeled "agree."

[b] p < .001.

implications for health delivery. Admission committees in medical schools have responded to pressures to choose students who at least voice a commitment to serve in geographic and specialty areas of need. If problems of maldistribution are to be remedied, then students will have to maintain their concern for patient needs, at least through four years of medical training.

Table 5.4 shows that most students (60.9) began medical school committed to choosing a specialty and geographic area that need physicians, although primary care and rural practice were more popular choices for meeting that commitment than inner-city ghetto practice. Among freshmen, most expected a primary-care career (72.8 percent) and rural practice (54.5 percent) to be at least somewhat likely, compared with only 24 percent that envisioned some possibility of an inner-city ghetto practice. Feeling a commitment to practice in patient-need areas poses students with a moral dilemma of choosing between their own needs and social responsibility. Rural practice may be a more satisfactory compromise to these students than inner-city medicine. Freshmen's commitment to patient need is consistent with the idealism they expressed in terms of helping others.

Compared with national data on medical students entering school in 1975, the same year respondents in this study began, students in North Carolina were considerably more interested in primary-care medicine. About 73 percent of the freshmen in the present study chose primary-care fields (family practice, internal medicine, and pediatrics)* compared with about 49 percent of the 1975 freshmen nationwide.[7] The enthusiasm for primary care among freshmen respondents may be due to the primary-care emphasis of some North Carolina medical schools and to their selection of many students from rural areas. A correlation between rural background and interest in primary care has been documented previously.[8]

Despite some individual fluctuation, seniors as a group leave medical school less interested in geographic and specialty areas of patient need than when they started. Seniors were considerably less oriented to primary-care medicine (50.9 percent), rural practice (34.2 percent), inner-city ghetto practice (15.1 percent), and choosing a specialty and area that needs doctors (41.2 percent) than they were as freshmen (72.8 percent, 54.5 percent, 24.1 percent, and 60.9 percent, respectively). Although admission committees in these

---

*In an open-ended question, students were asked, "Which field do you think you actually will be working in ten years from now?" Of the 258 who responded, 73 percent chose either family practice, internal medicine, or pediatrics.

North Carolina medical schools have successfully chosen students who were committed to serve geographic and specialty areas of patient need, the experience of medical school appears to somewhat undermine students' service commitments.

Interviews with medical students and previous research suggest a number of reasons for the waning interest in primary-care fields. First, although medical administrators may try to encourage primary care, the teachers that students model themselves after are principally specialists. The message in medical school is that to be competent one must specialize. As one female student related, "There is definitely that pressure that you're not really a good doctor if you go into family medicine. Being a family physician is to know not much about a lot of things." Students are shown the mistakes made by primary-care doctors in rural areas, a lesson that brings up students' worst malpractice fears. Furthermore, medical training encourages dependence on modern hospital technology and interest in rare as opposed to chronic and common illness, training not compatible with a rural, primary-care practice. Coupled with personal considerations (like wanting to work fewer hours and not wanting to be isolated), socialization in medical school seems to discourage patient-need practices.

Although students became less interested in primary-care and rural practices, medical administrators initiated many programs to help maintain students' interests in these practices. Family medicine rotations, special courses, and required programs where students work in rural areas have all been implemented to encourage rural and primary-care careers. Unfortunately, much of the medical training by housestaff and faculty seems to run counter to these administrators' goals.

Although there appears to be some pressure to specialize in medical school, not all types of primary-care practices have been discouraged to the same extent. The percentage distributions on three questionnaire items that ask seniors to evaluate whether faculty and housestaff encourage or discourage primary-care, family, and specialty practices are shown in Table 5.5. Twenty-two percent felt primary care was discouraged; about 36 percent felt family practice was discouraged; and about 5 percent felt specialty practice was discouraged. Thus, there seems to be somewhat more stigma attached to family practice than the other primary-care fields. Consistent with this finding, when freshmen were asked in which field they would be working, 50 percent said family practice, 8 percent indicated pediatrics, 14 percent chose internal medicine, and 27 percent said other fields. As seniors, only 16 percent chose family practice, 9 percent indicated pediatrics, fully 33 percent selected internal medi-

TABLE 5.5

Percentage Distributions of Senior Medical Students' Evaluations of
Whether Housestaff and Faculty Have Encouraged or Discouraged
Primary-Care, Family, and Specialty Practices, 1978

	Primary Care	Family Practice	Specialty Practice
Greatly discourage	2.5	7.9	0.0
Somewhat discourage	19.4	27.7	4.7
Neither encourage or discourage	30.9	29.1	32.0
Somewhat encourage	31.7	24.1	46.0
Greatly encourage	15.5	11.2	17.3
Total	100.0	100.0	100.0
Number	278	278	278

Note: Exact questions read, "To what extent do the faculty and
housestaff at your school encourage students to choose: (1) primary-
care practice, (2) family practice, and (3) specialty practice."

cine, and 42 percent said other fields. * Over time students tended to
select specialty practice, and those who stayed in primary-care fields
moved away from family practice and toward internal medicine. For
those interested in primary-care fields, internal medicine has probably seemed like a safer choice, since family practice is a new program with low prestige and is more subject to questions about the
adequacy of the training.

Table 5.4 shows that 34 percent and 15 percent of the seniors
expressed that they were at least somewhat likely to choose rural
practice and inner-city ghetto practice, respectively. When asked
the type of location in which they would most likely work, only about
14 percent said a rural area, and less than 1 percent chose an inner-
city ghetto location. Most seniors (60.3 percent) felt that a medium

*The field choices freshman year are based on 258 cases, and
in senior year on 276 cases. Those who did not know their field
choice have been excluded from the percentages. Freshman-year
percentages do not add to 100 percent due to rounding.

or small city (under 250,000) would be their most likely choice. * If North Carolina medical students are any indication of national trends, it seems likely that geographic maldistribution of physicians will continue to be a major health problem. Although there is a trend toward specialization in medical school, there still appears to be a substantial number of seniors interested in primary-care practice, especially internal medicine.

DISCUSSION AND SUMMARY

Some previous studies have implied that students do not lose their long-term idealistic perspective, that is, their desire to help people and their ideal view of medicine. [9] Others suggest that more encompassing cynical and attitudinal changes occur. [10] The present study tends to support the latter contention. Although most students maintained a general humanistic idealism, they were more realistic about physicians' limitations. General values of helping people did not indicate much social concern because by their senior year students became less willing to make personal sacrifices for patient need and less likely to advocate reforms of the medical profession that would aid poor and working-class Americans. Furthermore, despite most students' continuing denial of personal interest in money, many became considerably more critical of lowering physicians' incomes. Although students did not finish medical school with homogeneous opinions, on the whole they came closer to adopting traditional professional views, that is, political and economic status quo in the organization of medicine and geographic and specialty choice based on personal and professional interests rather than patient need. Students, however, should not be viewed as sponges accepting all dominant ideologies. For example, they retained concern with humanizing doctor/patient interactions even though few felt that faculty had been good role models in this respect.

So far the author has assumed that the reported changes in professional values and expectations have been the result of professional socialization in medical school. Discussions in the next chapter delve deeper into the issue of professional socialization with the testing of various explanations for why these orientation changes may have occurred over time. Some alternate explanations for the changes

---

*These data are based on 277 responses to the question, "Please circle the type of location you are most likely to work in: rural area, medium or small city (under 250,000), suburb of a large city, large city (nonghetto), large city (inner-city ghetto area)."

in professional orientations, such as maturation, are considered in the next as well as the concluding chapter.

To conclude, many students began medical school with a somewhat liberal and idealistic orientation on many issues concerning the practice and profession of medicine. The data presented in this chapter have illustrated that medical students generally became more conservative on political and economic issues in the profession and less concerned with patient needs in terms of geographic and specialty choices during medical training. Most respondents are not expected to push for major reforms in the medical profession, although many may serve in specialty areas of need. In addition, many students may establish humanitarian and egalitarian relationships with patients once they enter practice if values have any indications for future behavior. Seniors have more definite opinions on issues concerning sexism in medicine than they did as freshmen, although these changes have not resulted in more concern for women's causes. The impetus for changing the prejudicial treatment of women physicians and patients is not likely to come from students as a whole.

Most of these changes in professional orientations do not seem surprising considering the generally conservative atmosphere of most medical schools, with their emphasis on specialization and professional control over health care and their lack of attention to geographic maldistribution, rising medical costs, and sex discrimination. Furthermore, it seems that students' initial desires to choose patient-need practices have been somewhat undermined by training that has encouraged dependence on modern hospital technology, interest in rare diseases, and specialization as a way to avoid incompetence. If future doctors are going to be concerned with many of our present health-care problems, then it is the responsibility of medical educators to reexamine their dominant values and career priorities. It is a token gesture for admission committees to select students who are concerned with existing health-care problems if medical education not only does not reinforce their social service goals but appears to thwart them as well.

NOTES

1. Howard S. Becker, Blanche Geer, Everette C. Hughes, and Anselm L. Strauss, Boys in White (Chicago: University of Chicago Press, 1961), pp. 67-79; Samuel Bloom, Power and Dissent in the Medical School (New York: Free Press, 1973), pp. 75-107; Don Cahalan, Patricia Collette, and Norman A. Hilmar, "Career Interests and Expectations of U.S. Medical Students," Journal of Medical Education 32 (August 1957): 557-63; and Rodney M. Coe, Max Pepper,

and Mary Mattis, "The 'New' Medical Student: Another View," Journal of Medical Education 52 (February 1977): 89-98.

2. Leonard Eron, "The Effect of Medical Education on Attitudes: A Follow-up Study," Journal of Medical Education 33, pt. 2 (1958): 25-33; Leonard V. Gordon and Ivan N. Mensh, "Values of Medical School Students at Different Levels of Training," Journal of Educational Psychology 53 (1962): 48-50; Isabel R. Juan, Rosalia E. A. Paiva, Harold B. Haley, and Robert O'Keefe, "High and Low Levels of Dogmatism in Relation to Personality Characteristics of Medical Students: A Follow-up Study," Psychological Reports 34 (1974): 303-15; and Pearl P. Rosenberg, "Catch 22—The Medical Model," in Becoming a Physician, ed. Eileen C. Shapiro and Leah M. Lowenstein (Cambridge, Mass.: Ballinger, 1979), pp. 81-91.

3. Coe, Pepper, and Mattis, "The 'New' Medical Student," pp. 89-98; and Daniel Funkenstein, Medical Students, Medical Schools and Society during Five Eras: Factors Affecting the Career Choices of Physicians 1958-1976 (Cambridge, Mass.: Ballinger, 1978), pp. 83-103.

4. Becker et al., Boys in White, pp. 67-79; Bloom, Power and Dissent, pp. 93-107; Cahalan, Collette, and Hilmar, "Career Interests and Expectations," pp. 557-63.

5. Coe, Pepper, and Mattis, "The 'New' Medical Student," pp. 89-98.

6. Bloom, Power and Dissent, pp. 93-107.

7. The percentage choosing primary-care fields included those selecting family practice, internal medicine, and pediatrics among 1975 freshmen who had decided on a field. The percentages were calculated so that the undecided freshmen and those with no opinion were excluded from the total. See W. F. Dubé, Descriptive Study of Enrolled Medical Students 1975-76 (Washington, D.C.: Association of American Medical Colleges, 1977), pp. 67-68.

8. Richard Oates and Harry Feldman, "Patterns of Change in Medical Student Career Choices," Journal of Medical Education 49 (June 1974): 562-69.

9. Becker et al., Boys in White, pp. 67-79, 419-33; Juan et al., "High and Low Levels of Dogmatism," pp. 303-15; and Philip Perricone, "Social Concern in Medical Students: A Reconsideration of the Eron Assumption," Journal of Medical Education 49 (June 1974): 541-46.

10. Eron, "Effect of Medical Education on Attitudes," pp. 25-33; and Robert K. Merton, George G. Reader, and Patricia Kendall, eds., The Student-Physician (Cambridge, Mass.: Harvard University Press, 1957).

6

EXPLAINING CHANGES
IN PROFESSIONAL ORIENTATIONS

In the previous chapter, medical students were shown to become generally more conservative on political and economic issues in medicine, less interested in patient-need practices, and more realistic about physicians' limitations during their medical training. This chapter will focus on why these changes and individual fluctuations in professional orientations occur from first to last year in training, paying particular attention to the role of medical school experiences.

Most studies reporting attitudinal, personality, or value changes during medical school attribute these phenomena to professional socialization. Although not specified or tested, the experience of going through the rigors of medical training is assumed to cause great personal change. Rather than make such assumptions, the author has attempted to empirically discover what it is about the experience of medical school that results in some students changing and others maintaining their professional orientations. Furthermore, in explaining orientation change such factors as personality and numerous personal considerations were ignored so that the effect of schooling could be the main focus.

Before constructing the senior-year questionnaire, the author reviewed the professional socialization literature and conducted interviews with medical students to find clues for why medical training might have a transforming and generally conservative effect on students and why students seemed somewhat differentially affected by the experience. The interviews yielded the following diverse explanations for why orientations on practice and professional issues may have changed or remained stable over time: (1) anger at the way patients were treated by physicians; (2) good faculty and housestaff role models; (3) membership in a minority; (4) participation in liberal or minority groups and organizations; (5) interest in primary-care medicine that is more community oriented; (6) the conservative atmosphere of medical school and the medical profession; (7) conservatism among faculty and attending physicians; (8) the long hours, hard work, and general deprivation associated with medical training; (9) large medical school debts; (10) more information and more maturity by senior year; (11) ideological support from peers; and (12) exposure to the women's movement.

Students mentioned the first five factors listed above as helpful in either sustaining or changing to a liberal view. The second five factors were considered conducive to sustaining or developing conservatism. The last two factors—having ideological support from peers and exposure to the women's movement—could have either a conservative or liberal effect depending on the ideological position of one's friends and one's reaction to the women's movement and to women espousing these views. For some, especially the men, exposure to the women's movement seemed to result in a conservative backlash of opinion toward women's causes. This backlash effect will be discussed in Chapter 7.

The reasons provided by students for stability and change on professional orientations along with some other possible explanations, including measures of students' background characteristics, were tested using multiple regression techniques in a model of professional orientation change. Therefore, the main focus of this chapter is the analysis of how experiences in medical school and background characteristics affect students' orientations. Issues will be explored such as whether agreeing with faculty and feeling deprived due to the long work hours might lead to greater conservatism during medical training.

The path model shown in Figure 6.1 presents the theoretical ordering of the variables with an exact list of all the variables tested. The utility of the model of professional orientation change depends on the validity of the theory indicating the causal sequence among variables. Interviews with medical students and logical considerations provided reasonable support for the causal order of variables in the model. Background characteristics (for example, race and sex) were placed first in the model because these were fixed at birth or at least during childhood. Although experiences in medical school were measured in the senior year at the same time follow-up data on professional orientations were gathered, these experiences in school were assumed to occur prior to senior-year orientations. Issues brought up in student interviews suggested that school experiences, especially in the clinical years of training, resulted in professional orientation change. In some specific cases it probably can be argued that the relationship between orientation and experience is reciprocal. Instances where causal order appears questionable will be noted in the

FIGURE 6.1

Causal Model for Explaining Change in Professional Orientations from Freshman to Senior Year

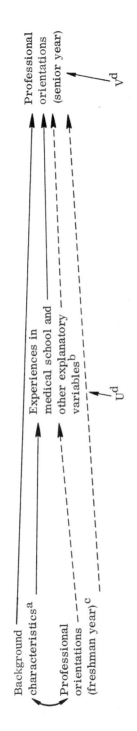

[a]Background characteristics include sex, race, father's education, age, religion, and rural-to-urban origins.

[b]Experiences in medical school and other explanatory variables include marital status, parental status (having children), medical school being attended, grades, medical school debts, student treated badly, patients treated badly, viewing career negatively, experiencing school difficulty, supporting women's movement, being active in liberal organizations, disagreeing with faculty, becoming more conservative, getting ideological support from peers, planning academic medicine career in senior year (except with predicting change in primary-care plans), planning primary-care career in senior year (except with predicting change in primary-care plans), and school encouraging primary care (only with physician maldistribution issues).

[c]To measure change in professional orientations, professional orientations at time 1 were used to predict orientations at time 2. Thus, the professional orientations at time 1 were entered into the equations first, before the background variables. Since the professional orientations freshman year operate as control variables, the arrows in the figure for these variables are broken. The professional orientations include all those previously considered, which are listed in Tables 6.2, 6.4, 6.6, and 6.8.

[d]U and V are residual variables, that is, variables not in the model, which also might explain variation.

discussion of the findings. For the most part, however, experiences in medical school would seem to occur prior to the development of one's senior-year professional orientations.

The best way to analyze change in longitudinal research has been a long-debated controversy among statisticians.[1] Although subtracting the orientation scores at time 1 from time 2 would seem the most intuitive approach, these change scores are systematically related to any random measurement error. Thus, change scores may reflect unreliability of the measures more than any real change. In order to avoid change scores, a regressed change analysis was used,[2] that is, each professional orientation measured freshman year was entered first into the equation predicting that orientation at time two before other explanatory variables. By controlling on initial orientation, we can assess the relative importance of explanatory variables (for example, students' backgrounds and experiences in medical school) in explaining professional orientation change. This regressed change analysis also lets us judge the importance of particular explanatory variables in predicting professional orientation change while controlling for the effects of all the intervening variables simultaneously. Thus, we can assess the independent effect of each explanatory variable net of other variables in the model.

The full equations for predicting professional orientation change included all the variables listed in the first two footnotes in Figure 6.1. Because many of the explanatory variables did not significantly contribute to explaining variation in professional orientation change, these equations were rerun with only the significant explanatory variables included. For the most part, the standardized regression coefficients in the shortened or truncated equations closely approximated the coefficients in the long equations. In cases where a regression coefficient in the truncated model was greatly suppressed or was much larger than in the long equations, the explanatory variable(s) causing these effects were added to the shortened equations. The resulting truncated equations explained approximately the same percentage of variation in change as the full model and the regression coefficients in the shortened equations were approximately equal to those in the longer model. It is important to remember that the interpretation of the results did not differ in the truncated versions and that random measurement error could easily account for the slight differences between the regression coefficients in the long versus the short equations. The shortened results allow for a clearer and less cluttered presentation of the findings.

Tables 6.2, 6.4, 6.6, and 6.8 show the standardized and unstandardized regression coefficients in the shortened equations for a model of professional orientation change with R^2 (explained variance) and constant for each equation. The unstandardized regression coefficient indicates how much the dependent variable changes with one unit change in the predictor variable. Because the standardized regression coefficient indicates the change in the dependent variable (in standard deviation units) for every one standard deviation change in the predictor variable, this standardized score facilitates comparisons among variables with different ranges. In the present model, the standardized coefficients indicate the importance of each predictor variable in explaining change over time while controlling the effects of the other same or prior stage variables. The effects of explanatory variables will be small in cases where there was little individual or group change over time, because these instances do not provide much variation to explain.[*]

Tables 6.1, 6.3, 6.5, and 6.7 show the means on freshman- and senior-year professional orientations by students' background characteristics. The orientations considered in these four tables correspond to the four health-care problem areas respectively, that is, physicians' relationships with patients, political and economic change, the treatment of women physicians and patients, and physician maldistribution. These tables have been included to aid the interpretation of the findings concerning professional orientation change. Understanding differential changes in professional orientations over time can be facilitated by examining how students' backgrounds (for example, race, sex, and social class) affect their initial orientations. Thus, for example, if blacks did not become as conservative over time on a particular issue, it would be useful to know where they started and finished in relation to whites. Furthermore, the significant freshman orientation differences among students of different backgrounds for the most part persisted while controlling on other background characteristics. In other words, almost all of the significant freshman orientation differences reported in Tables 6.1, 6.3, 6.5, and 6.7 cannot be attributed to differences on other background characteristics. The few cases where significant background differences did not hold after controlling on other background variables have been reported in the text.

Briefly, by examing Tables 6.1, 6.3, 6.5, and 6.7, we see that sex followed closely by father's educational attainment are the best background predictors of students' initial orientations. Sex dif-

---

[*]The zero-order correlation matrix between explanatory variables and professional orientations was not considered helpful with interpreting a regressed change analysis so it was not included in the text. Chapter 3 gives the means and standard deviations for the variables concerning experiences in medical school.

ferences on professional orientations initially and over time are the
focus of Chapters 7 and 8; this chapter will only briefly discuss the
findings related to how men and women change differently during their
medical training.

PHYSICIANS' RELATIONSHIPS WITH PATIENTS

Changes in the professional values and expectations of medical students from their first to last year in school were detailed in
the previous chapter. On most values concerning the doctor/patient
relationship, students as a group changed little, although there was
some individual fluctuation over time. The exception to this trend
was that students became considerably more critical of physicians'
expertise.

Table 6.2 shows which explanatory variables appear to explain
changes in students' orientations concerning the doctor/patient relationship from freshman to senior year. With this table and Table 6.1,
we can examine the role that students' background characteristics
have played in regard to changing opinions about physicians' relationships with patients. To begin, females were more likely during their
training to realize the importance of providing health information
to patients and the importance of patients being critical of physicians'
judgments (including physicians criticizing each other in public). In
contrast, blacks—another minority group in medicine—began school
slightly (although not significantly) more oriented than whites to providing health information to patients but finished slightly less interested in this patient-care issue (see Table 6.1). Race, however,
appeared unimportant in explaining attitudinal change on other patient-
care orientations.

Students' religious backgrounds appear somewhat important in
predicting orientation change on issues concerning physicians' relationships with patients. Table 6.1 indicates that, when compared
with students from other religious groups and no religious preference,
Jewish respondents began school more in favor of patients being critical of physicians' judgments and they finished even more critical
than others of physicians' expertise. Although all students became
more critical over time, being Jewish tended to further a more critical evaluation of physicians' limitations. In addition, whereas Protestant and Catholic students maintained about the same degree of interest in social and psychological factors in health care from freshman to senior year, Jewish students became slightly more committed
to these humanistic patient-care ideals. Furthermore, Table 6.2
shows that those with no religious affiliation (the omitted category
under religion) became less interested in the social and psychological

TABLE 6.1

Means on Freshman and Senior Professional Orientations concerning Physicians' Relationships with Patients by Students' Background Characteristics

Freshman/Senior Year (range of values). Each cell shows Freshman (top) / Senior (bottom).

Professional Orientations	Sex: Male	Sex: Female	Race: White	Race: Black	Religion: Protestant	Religion: Catholic	Religion: Jewish	Religion: None	Background: Rural	Background: Small Town	Background: Suburb, Medium City	Background: Medium City	Background: Suburb, Large City	Background: Large City	Age[a] (freshman year): 23 or Less	Age[a]: 24 or More	Father's Education[a]: College or Less	Father's Education[a]: More than College
Give health information (1–5)	3.25 / 3.24	3.34 / 3.48[b]	3.25 / 3.31	3.53 / 3.10	3.27 / 3.32	3.21 / 3.23	3.55 / 3.49	2.64 / 2.71	3.15 / 3.33	3.19 / 3.32	3.46 / 3.21	3.19 / 3.24	3.53 / 3.41	3.29 / 3.20	3.28 / 3.26	3.29 / 3.48[c]	3.20 / 3.23	3.36[b] / 3.39[b]
Critical of doctors (1–5)	2.78 / 3.29	2.93 / 3.55[b]	2.83 / 3.36	2.79 / 3.58	2.74 / 3.32	2.90 / 3.14	3.40 / 4.09	2.86[b] / 3.29[c]	2.50 / 3.33	2.75 / 3.19	2.83 / 3.43	2.81 / 3.35	3.17 / 3.72	2.83[b] / 3.24	2.80 / 3.27	2.89 / 3.67[b]	2.70 / 3.27	2.97[c] / 3.48
Social/psychological important (1–5)	4.25 / 4.27	4.54[c] / 4.50[c]	4.34 / 4.32	4.22 / 4.42	4.32 / 4.30	4.32 / 4.36	4.29 / 4.52	4.62 / 4.10	4.15 / 4.21	4.40 / 4.40	4.42 / 4.43	4.29 / 4.29	4.23 / 4.28	4.52 / 4.30	4.32 / 4.31	4.32 / 4.41	4.30 / 4.29	4.35 / 4.38
Helping people important (1–4)	3.31 / 3.11	3.45[b] / 3.19	3.34 / 3.10	3.32 / 3.28	3.38 / 3.19	3.24 / 2.98	3.13 / 3.04	3.43 / 2.47[c]	3.43 / 3.18	3.32 / 3.12	3.35 / 3.36	3.32 / 3.05	3.27 / 3.04	3.62 / 3.32	3.34 / 3.15	3.34 / 3.08	3.36 / 3.14	3.32 / 3.11
Number of cases	207	72	247	24	208	39	23	7	36	85	23	64	48	21	213	60	160	119

[a]For readability the interval variables, age and father's education, were each grouped into two categories. Age has been divided into 23 or less at the beginning of school and 24 or more at the onset of school. Father's education has been divided into college degree or less and more than a college degree. The tests of significance for the correlations of age and father's education with professional values and expectations were computed on the ungrouped data. The grouped data represent a rough approximation of the age and father's education effects.

[b]p < .05.

[c]p < .01.

113

TABLE 6.2

Standardized and Unstandardized Regression Coefficients for a Model of Professional Orientation Change concerning Doctor/Patient Relationships

(with R^2 and constant for each equation)

Freshman-Year Professional Orientations and Explanatory Variables	Senior-Year Professional Orientations			
	Standardized Coefficients		Unstandardized Coefficients	
Give Health Information				
Give health information	.423[a]		.418[a]	
Sex[c]	.412[a]	.321[a]	.406[a]	.316[a]
Race[c]	.134[b]	.101	.238[b]	.178
Age	-.110[b]	-.148[b]	-.300[b]	-.403
	.129[b]	.117[b]	.053[b]	.048[b]
School				
Duke		.169[b]		.281[b]
University of North Carolina		.218[a]		.342[a]
Experience school difficulty		-.144[b]		-.122[b]
Disagree with faculty		.130[b]		.161[b]
Support women's movement		.137[b]		.129[b]
Active in liberal organizations		.006		.006
Academic medicine plans (senior)		-.113		-.101
R^2	.179	.306		
Constant	.224	.572	1.932	.531
Critical of Doctors				
Critical of doctors	.433[a]	.357[a]	.406[a]	.334[a]
Sex	.393[a]	-.005	.368[a]	-.013
	.130[b]		.299[b]	
Religion[d]				
Protestant		.062		.144
Catholic		-.067		-.193
Jewish		.161		.587
Age		.061		.032
School debts		.130[b]		.012[b]
Support women's movement		.246[a]		.300[a]
Disagree with faculty		.193[a]		.312[a]
R^2	.188	.363		
Constant	.246	.288	2.216	-.375

114

				Social/Psychological Important		
Social/psychological important	.366[a]	.353[a]	.360[a]	.385[a]	.372[a]	.380[a]
Religion						
Protestant		.177	.146		.234	.193
Catholic		.171[b]	.155		.283	.257
Jewish		.238[b]	.215[b]		.497[b]	.447[b]
Sex		.110	.114[b]		.144	.150[b]
Race		.078	.050		.157	.101
School						
Duke			.115			.142
University of North Carolina			.231[a]			.268[a]
R^2	.134	.169	.203			
Constant			2.661	2.411	2.262	

				Helping People Important		
Helping people important	.428[a]	.427[a]	.340[a]	.464[a]	.463[a]	.369[a]
Religion						
Protestant		.441[a]	.405[a]		.637[a]	.584[a]
Catholic		.277[b]	.299[a]		.500[b]	.540[a]
Jewish		.269[a]	.290[a]		.612[a]	.661[a]
Experience school difficulty			.208[a]			.143[a]
Primary-care plans (senior)			.300[a]			.124[a]
View career negatively			-.193[a]			-.110[a]
R^2	.183	.216	.363			
Constant			1.578	.984	.735	

R^2 = multiple correlation

[a] $p \leq .01$.

[b] $p \leq .05$.

[c] Sex and race are coded so that males and whites equal zero and females and blacks equal one, respectively. All other variables are coded so that a high score indicates high on the variables as labeled.

[d] School and religion have been recoded into dummy variables. The omitted variable of the three school variables is Bowman Gray. The omitted variable of the four religion variables is "no religious affiliation." The regression coefficients for both omitted categories (Bowman Gray and no religious affiliation) are equal to zero.

aspects of patient care and in helping people than Protestant, Catholic, or Jewish students.* It seems that having a religious affiliation furthers humanistic patient-care values, especially among Jewish students.

Finally, among the background factors, age appears to have some relevance for change on egalitarian patient-care values. Table 6.1 indicates that young and old students begin school with similar professional orientations, but older respondents were somewhat more likely to leave school recognizing the importance of informing patients about diagnosis and disease and supporting patients' critical appraisals of physicians. Thus, over time being either older, Jewish, or female (minority statuses in medical school) seems to further more egalitarian doctor/patient values (that is, views contrary to mainstream medicine).

As mentioned in the previous chapter, most school differences in professional orientations during freshman year were explained by variations in students' social background characteristics, that is, they were mostly a function of students' differing backgrounds. Because the freshman questionnaire was administered during the first week of school, school differences that year reflected self-selection and/or school selection policies. Changes in orientation associated with the school one attended can be thought of as reflecting some experience or factor that differed among the schools. Thus, the author does not place much importance on senior-year school differences; because these are proxies for other (unmeasured) experiences that have varied at the schools.

To summarize school differences briefly, Table 6.2 shows that after controlling on background variables, Bowman Gray students were slightly less likely than students at the other two schools to maintain their commitment to giving patients health information concerning diagnosis and illness. (Bowman Gray is the omitted category with a regression coefficient equal to zero compared with .169 and .218 at Duke and UNC respectively.) In addition, those at the University of North Carolina were slightly more likely to increase their interest

---

*The regression coefficients for any omitted category of a dummy variable (for example, school and religion) are equal to zero, which facilitates comparisons between these variables and other categories of the dummy variables. For example, Table 6.2 shows that Protestant (.441), Catholic (.277) and Jewish (.269) students were more likely to maintain interest in helping people than those with no religious affiliation (0) (standardized regression coefficients reported in parentheses).

in social and psychological factors in health care. This might reflect differences in the socialization experiences of those students. After controlling on other explanatory variables, the school one attends did not appear to explain any other changes in professional values pertaining to doctor/patient interactions.

Disagreement with medical school faculty and attending physicians' political medical views and familiarity or support of the women's movement were important predictors of egalitarian views toward patients (note the first two professional orientations in Table 6.2). Specifically, from freshman to senior year those who supported the women's movement and those who disagreed with the faculty's views tended to maintain a greater emphasis on giving health information to patients and tended to develop even more critical views toward physicians' expertise than students more accepting of faculty and less familar with the women's movement. Because traditionally the medical school faculty and attending physicians have been role models for less egalitarian doctor/patient relationships, it is not surprising to find less authoritarian values among those students who reject such role models and likewise more authoritarian values among those who accept their mentors. Because the women's movement and the women's health literature has emphasized the need for more egalitarian treatment of women patients, this philosophy seems to have carried over to all patients. Thus, rejecting traditional role models and replacing them with alternative ideologies (for example, the women's movement) appears to encourage less elitist professional values.

Two other variables have a small role in predicting change in egalitarian patient-care values: difficulty in school and school debts. Table 6.2 indicates that those who experience the most difficulty in school in terms of the time pressures were slightly less likely to maintain their support for giving patients health information after controlling on other explanatory variables. Perhaps the time constraints of medical training make students less willing to invest effort in what they might feel are the "frills" of medicine. On the other hand, the larger one's debts in medical school, the more students became critical of patients accepting physicians' expertise.

Aside from the background variables, experiences in medical school (for the most part support of the women's movement and disagreeing with faculty) explained only about 8 percent and 12 percent of the change on the two orientations concerning egalitarian doctor/patient relationships. (These percentages refer to the change in R^2 when explanatory variables are added to equations predicting the first two professional orientations in Table 6.2.) Much of the change on these values remained unexplained by the path model. Interviews with medical students reported in the previous chapter suggested that students became more critical of physicians' expertise as they had more contact with actual medical practice.

Because there was not much variation in either freshman or senior year on the index concerning the importance of social and psychological factors in health care, it was not surprising that specific experiences in medical school did not explain change on this value. The little change that occurred on this index was probably mostly the result of random measurement error.

Whereas experiencing school difficulty in terms of time pressures seemed to promote slightly less egalitarian views, that is, less desire to give patients information, it also appeared to sustain students' idealistic concerns with helping people. These findings seem somewhat contradictory, although wanting to help people can be a patronizing rather than an egalitarian attitude. If feeling deprived maintains greater altruism, it may be that values of aiding mankind help students justify their time sacrifices. Interestingly, viewing one's career negatively led to less idealistic values over time (note coefficients in Table 6.2 concerning the value "helping people important"). Thus, feeling that one has worked hard was related to greater idealism, yet going so far as to believe that medicine was unenjoyable and was the wrong career choice resulted in less desire to help others.

As expected, those choosing primary-care medicine were much less likely to lose sight of the importance of helping others. It is unclear whether choosing primary care resulted in greater altruistic values or whether an orientation to helping others aided in sustaining a commitment to primary care. The latter interpretation seems like a better explanation of this finding.

POLITICAL AND ECONOMIC CHANGE
IN THE MEDICAL PROFESSION

In Chapter 5, we saw that students tended to become more conservative on political and economic change issues in medicine. Table 6.4 shows that few student background characteristics explain these conservative value shifts. During the senior year, women were slightly less likely than men to lose their liberal stance on the issue of reducing the profession's control over health care and yet slightly more likely to reduce their time commitment to volunteer work. As shown in Table 6.3, females began and finished medical school with more liberal values on most political and economic change issues.

Black students were more likely than whites to start school advocating government intervention to reduce professional control over health care and planning both volunteer service and political and social change work in medicine (see Table 6.3). Blacks remained

TABLE 6.3

Means on Freshman and Senior Professional Orientations concerning Political and Economic Change in the Medical Profession by Students' Background Characteristics

Freshman/Senior Year (range of values). Each cell shows freshman value / senior value.

Professional Orientations	Sex Male	Sex Female	Race White	Race Black	Religion Protestant	Religion Catholic	Religion Jewish	Religion None	Background Rural	Background Small Town	Background Suburb, Medium City	Background Medium City	Background Suburb, Large City	Background Large City	Age[a] 23 or Less	Age[a] 24 or More	Father's Education[a] College or Less	Father's Education[a] More than College
Reduce profession's control (1–5)	2.88 / 2.41	3.19[b] / 2.90[c]	2.89 / 2.45	3.56[c] / 3.35[c]	2.83 / 2.46	3.11 / 2.58	3.75 / 3.26	2.91[c] / 2.74[c]	2.88 / 2.48	2.79 / 2.36	2.90 / 2.66	3.11 / 2.76	3.14 / 2.55	3.00 / 2.50	3.00 / 2.54	2.92 / 2.52	2.91 / 2.45	3.03 / 2.66[c]
Favor National Service Corps (1–3)	1.89 / 1.68	2.11[c] / 1.86[b]	1.95 / 1.73	1.83 / 1.67	1.91 / 1.69	2.00 / 1.77	1.91 / 1.91	1.86 / 1.86	1.72 / 1.72	1.98 / 1.68	1.78 / 1.70	1.92 / 1.70	2.15 / 1.83	2.00[b] / 1.76	1.95 / 1.74	1.98 / 1.70	1.88 / 1.69	2.04[c] / 1.78
No profits in health care (1–5)	2.85 / 2.28	3.33[c] / 2.78[c]	2.91 / 2.36	3.33 / 2.67	2.93 / 2.33	3.03 / 2.69	3.50 / 2.65	2.43 / 2.14	2.86 / 2.44	2.93 / 2.38	3.13 / 2.52	2.98 / 2.36	2.81 / 2.25	3.33 / 2.86	3.08 / 2.53	2.63[c] / 1.95[c]	2.95 / 2.38	3.01 / 2.45
Lower doctor income (1–5)	2.98 / 2.67	3.38[c] / 3.02[c]	3.09 / 2.77	3.01 / 2.70	3.00 / 2.72	3.28 / 2.80	3.38 / 3.13	3.00 / 2.64	2.84 / 2.67	2.87 / 2.72	3.16 / 2.80	3.18 / 2.86	3.33 / 2.83	3.32[c] / 2.70	3.08 / 2.77	3.11 / 2.73	2.97 / 2.64	3.23[c] / 2.93[c]
Income is important (1–4)	1.99 / 2.16	1.80[c] / 1.98[b]	1.94 / 2.10	2.06 / 2.30	1.98 / 2.14	1.89 / 2.12	1.70 / 1.92	1.96 / 2.00[b]	2.03 / 2.14	2.04 / 2.19	1.76 / 1.85	1.89 / 2.12	1.83 / 2.06	1.96 / 2.13	1.94 / 2.10	1.96 / 2.19	2.01 / 2.20	1.84 / 2.01[c]
Work for political change (1–4)	2.12 / 1.79	2.31[b] / 2.06[c]	2.12 / 1.82	2.71[c] / 2.22[c]	2.10 / 1.81	2.30 / 2.05	2.55 / 1.99	2.09[b] / 1.71	2.18 / 1.80	2.10 / 1.80	2.18 / 1.88	2.15 / 1.95	2.35 / 1.92	2.03 / 1.76	2.16 / 1.87	2.24 / 1.86	2.11 / 1.74	2.25 / 2.02[c]
Plan volunteer work (0–80)	17.09 / 11.92	18.74 / 9.91[b]	16.80 / 11.17	24.48[c] / 13.58	17.49 / 11.61	16.89 / 10.58	16.77 / 11.00	20.00 / 7.86	16.00 / 11.72	16.40 / 11.77	16.18 / 10.64	19.05 / 11.57	17.91 / 10.89	20.53 / 10.95	17.70 / 11.63	16.91 / 10.71	17.92 / 11.33	16.95 / 11.50
Number of cases[d]	207	72	247	24	208	39	23	7	36	85	23	64	48	21	213	60	160	119

[a] For readability the interval variables, age and father's education, were each grouped into two categories. Age has been divided into 23 or less at the beginning of school and 24 or more at the onset of school. Father's education has been divided into college degree or less and more than a college degree. The tests of significance for the correlations of age and father's education with professional values and expectations were computed on the ungrouped data. The grouped data represent a rough approximation of the age and father's education effects.

[b] p < .05.

[c] p < .01.

[d] Calculations are based on the number of cases shown except for the single-item measures (favor National Service Corps, no profits in health care, plan volunteer work), which are computed on slightly fewer cases.

TABLE 6.4

Standardized and Unstandardized Regression Coefficients for a Model of Professional Orientation Change concerning Political and Economic Change in the Medical Profession (with R^2 and constant for each equation)

Freshman-Year Professional Orientations and Explanatory Variables	Senior-Year Professional Orientations			
	Standardized Coefficients		Unstandardized Coefficients	
Reduce Profession's Control				
Reduce profession's control	.602[a]		.588[a]	
Sex[c]	.549[a]	.462[a]	.536[a]	.451[a]
Race[c]	.126[a]	.063	.288[a]	.145
Father's education	.171[a]	.243[a]	.600[a]	.854[a]
School[d]	.113[b]	.059	.030[b]	.016
Duke		.161[a]		.344[a]
University of North Carolina		.103		.209
Support women's movement		.262[a]		.318[a]
Active in liberal organizations		-.131[b]		-.155[b]
Become more conservative		-.196[a]		-.281[a]
R^2	.363	.414		.345
Constant	.510		.796	.044
Favor National Service Corps				
Favor National Service Corps	.371[a]		.401[a]	
R^2	.138			
Constant	.943			
No Profits in Health Care				
No profits in health care	.532[a]	.517[a]	.502[a]	.487[a]
Experience school difficulty		.145[b]		.186[a]
Disagree with faculty		.127[b]		.240[b]
R^2	.283			
Constant	.325		.913	-.315
Lower Doctor Income				
Lower doctor income	.629[a]	.635[a]	.654[a]	.659[a]
	.558[a]		.580[a]	
Urban background	-.119[b]	-.111[b]	-.066[b]	-.061[b]
Father's education	.116[b]	.073	.026[b]	.017

	(1)	(2)	(3)
School		.142[b]	.258[b]
Duke		.112[b]	.191[b]
University of North Carolina		.173[a]	.178[a]
Support women's movement	.396	.417	
R^2			.268
Constant			.459

Income Is Important

	(1)	(2)	(3)	(4)
Income is important	.571[a]	.534[a]	.568[a]	.531[a]
Support women's movement		-.193[a]		-.138[a]
R^2	.327		.530	.750
Constant		.362	1.015	1.458

Work for Political Change

	(1)	(2)	(3)	(4)	(5)	(6)
Work for political change	.570[a]	.560[a]	.563[a]	.554[a]	.414[a]	.409[a]
Father's education	.125[b]			.024[b]	.142[a]	.028[a]
School					.105	.164
Duke					.131[b]	.192[b]
University of North Carolina					.126[b]	.109[b]
Active in liberal organizations					.169[a]	.081[a]
Primary-care plans (senior)					.201[a]	.235[a]
Disagree with faculty						
R^2	.324	.340	.638	.271		
Constant					.448	-.724

Plan Volunteer Work

	(1)	(2)	(3)	(4)	(5)
Plan volunteer work	.477[a]	.486[a]	.327[a]	.333[a]	.333[a]
Sex	-.141[b]	-.174[a]		-2.549[b]	-3.142[a]
Experience school difficulty		.133[b]			1.156[b]
R^2	.228	.247			
Constant			5.669	6.221	2.793

[a] $p \le .01$.

[b] $p \le .05$.

[c] Sex and race are coded so that males and whites equal zero and females and blacks equal one. All other variables are coded so that a high score indicates high on the variable as labeled.

[d] School has been recoded into three dummy variables. The omitted variable is Bowman Gray, which has regression coefficients equal to zero.

more committed to most of these liberal professional values, especially to programs like socialized medicine to reduce professional control over health care. They did not, however, remain significantly more committed than whites to volunteer service.

Students from upper-socioeconomic-status homes (as indicated by their father's educational attainment) began school more favorable to lowering physicians' incomes and to a compulsory National Service Corps without remuneration (see Table 6.3). It makes sense that children from high-socioeconomic-status families can afford to be less concerned about the economic rewards associated with becoming a physician. As they went through school, these economically privileged students were also slightly more likely to retain their liberal values and expectations on some issues concerning political and economic change (for example, reducing the profession's control over health care, lowering doctors' incomes, and working for political change).

Upon entrance to medical school, those students from rural areas were less likely than those raised in cities to favor a compulsory National Service Corps for physicians and the lowering of physicians' incomes and status (see Table 6.3). The conservative effects of the socialization process appeared to wipe out these initial differences between rural and urban students.

As mentioned before, most of the school differences freshman year were explained by variations in students' backgrounds. The data in Table 6.4 show that Bowman Gray (the omitted school category) has a slightly more conservative impact on students' political and economic orientations that has not been accounted for by the measured school experiences. This was not surprising because students at Bowman Gray were more likely to rate their school conservative (51 percent) than students at Duke (41 percent) or the University of North Carolina (12 percent).*

The author initially predicted that not becoming more conservative in political outlook over time, being familiar with and supporting the women's movement, being active in liberal organizations, and disagreeing with faculty on political issues would lead to the maintenance of more liberal professional values and expectations. To some extent the data in Table 6.4 support these hypotheses. Those who supported the women's movement (regardless of their sex) were less likely to reject the lowering of physicians' incomes and govern-

---

*This question reads, "Overall, is the political atmosphere at your school: (1) liberal, (2) middle of the road, (3) conservative." (274 students responded to the item.)

ment intervention to reduce professional control over health care and more likely to deny personal interest in large incomes and status from first to last year in school. These findings make sense because the women's health literature presents a critical view of the political and economic structure of the medical profession, and supporting the women's movement is an indication of being more liberal and less traditional.

Activity in liberal and minority organizations did not contribute much to the maintenance of a liberal orientation (see Table 6.4). Although those who were active in liberal organizations in medical school remained more interested in working for political and social change, they were slightly less likely to remain committed to reducing the profession's control over health care. This latter finding seems confusing because those who were active in liberal and minority organizations both began and finished school with more liberal views concerning this issue of limiting professional autonomy. Liberal organizational affiliation contributes to conservative change more than nonparticipation only when controlling for the effects of race and sex; blacks and females are more likely to be members of minority and liberal organizations. When sex and race are not held constant, organizational affiliation actually contributes to more liberal change on the issue of professional autonomy. Thus, it is not organizational affiliation that helps maintain liberalism, but being female and/or black that is important. Therefore, it can be concluded that activity in liberal and minority organizations for the most part did not appear to prevent or promote conservative change on political and economic issues in medicine.[*]

Table 6.4 indicates that from freshman to senior year, those who became more conservative in their general political outlook were somewhat more likely to reject such programs as socialized medicine to reduce the professions's control over health care. Becoming more politically conservative from first to last year, however, did not contribute to any other conservative changes on political and economic

---

*The finding that liberal organizational affiliation contributes to conservative change more than nonparticipation is in part an artifact of measurement; that is, those active in such organizations start out so high on the liberal scales that they have nowhere to go but down. Other students scoring in the middle range on this issue of reducing professional control over health care can change in both directions, that is, by becoming more or less liberal. Owing to the problem of high scorers tending to regress toward the mean, interpretation of such findings must be reevaluated.

issues in medicine. Thus, there was little support for the contention that growing conservatism on medical issues is a reflection of the increasing political conservatism of the decade.

Disagreeing with faculty and attending physicians on political issues promoted slightly more opposition to hospitals, drug companies, and insurance companies making profits on health care and considerably more commitment to work for political change in medicine (see Table 6.4). Likewise, it appears that the students who accepted faculty and attending physicians' views were conservatively influenced by their role models.

During interviews with students, some mentioned interest in primary care as a factor contributing to their more liberal professional views. As shown in Table 6.4, interest in primary care tends to promote more commitment to working for political and social change in medicine. Because primary care is a somewhat deviant although much needed career choice in medicine today, those who select these fields have demonstrated greater social concern and commitment to change than students in the mainstream of medicine.

Originally, the author proposed that students who experienced difficulty in school might become more conservative as a result of feeling deprived. As one female at Bowman Gray explained,

> After going through that third year and seeing what its going to be like and seeing the long hours, I think most of the students in our class want to feel financially paid for their efforts. I'm not saying they all want to go out and make $200,000 a year but they all want to be secure if they have to work that hard. They do want to be paid for it.

Contrary to expectation, students who felt that medical school had been difficult due to the time demands were more likely to remain opposed to excessive profits made in health care and to continue to plan volunteer work (see Table 6.4). Furthermore, those who felt that medical school was difficult were not more likely to be concerned with the financial rewards of medicine. The correlations between experiencing school difficulty and expressing interest in money and favoring lower physician incomes were insignificant. Deprivation, at least during medical school, has not been shown to contribute to more conservative or economically acquisitive views, but rather to less traditional views and more humanitarian plans. Furthermore, the author had expected to find that high medical school debts would also lead to more conservative economic values in medicine, but this did not happen.

Variations on background characteristics and school experiences accounted for relatively little of the change on most professional orientations concerning political and economic issues in medicine. (Table 6.4 shows that explained variance, R^2, ranged from zero to 15 percent after subtracting the R^2 of the professional orientations at time 1.) The conservative nature of medical training, of the medical profession, and of the medical school faculty would seem to be the best explanation of students' growing conservatism. One need only look at the publications of drug companies and the American Medical Association to realize the conservative stands that the profession and related arms of the American health empire take on such issues as government intervention in health care. As mentioned in Chapter 5, few medical students rate the political atmosphere of their school as liberal, most indicating either middle of the road or conservative. As one female at Bowman Gray suggested,

> You learn things by experience and the experience of people you see around you. The people [medical school faculty] we see are for the most part fairly conservative. There are some who are liberal clear out to the ends. . . . But for the most part. . .the people you hang around rubs off on you and these people are very conservative and some of their conservative values have probably rubbed off on us.

In interviews with medical students many expressed similar sentiments about the conservative atmosphere of medical school (see Chapter 5). Those students, however, who remained committed to alternative reference groups (for example, the women's movement) and those who rejected their role models' views tended to be better equipped to resist the conservative impact of medical training.

PREJUDICE AGAINST WOMEN PHYSICIANS AND PATIENTS

Change on issues concerning discrimination toward women physicians and patients has been characterized by individual and subgroup fluctuation rather than by attitudinal shifts in the group as a whole. In other words, the stability of the means over time on most of these indexes has tended to mask the fact that many individuals have either become more or less concerned with prejudice toward women. Table 6.6 shows that much of the change on women's issues can be explained by the students' gender, being dissatisfied with the way patients were treated, and being familiar with and supporting the women's movement.

Table 6.5 shows that women medical students began school more aware than men of the problems faced by women in medicine. Further-

TABLE 6.5

Means on Freshman and Senior Professional Orientations concerning the Treatment of Women Physicians and Patients by Students' Background Characteristics

Freshman/Senior Year (range of values)

Professional Orientations	Sex Male	Sex Female	Race White	Race Black	Religion Protestant	Religion Catholic	Religion Jewish	Religion None	Background Rural	Background Small Town	Background Suburb, Medium City	Background Medium City	Background Suburb, Large City	Background Large City	Age[a] (freshman year) 23 or Less	Age[a] 24 or More	Father's Education[a] College or Less	Father's Education More than College
Bias toward women doctors (1–5)	2.95 / 2.87	3.14 / 3.05	2.99 / 2.93	3.18 / 2.96	3.02 / 2.91	2.79 / 2.96	3.15 / 2.91	3.21 / 3.29	2.95 / 2.93	3.02 / 2.91	3.22 / 3.17	2.98 / 2.93	3.08 / 2.93	2.62 / 2.60	3.04 / 2.94	2.84 / 2.85	3.00 / 2.90	2.99 / 2.94
Specialty choice pressure on women (1–5)	3.08 / 2.95	3.54[b] / 3.75[b]	3.20 / 3.13	3.25 / 3.63[c]	3.19 / 3.16	3.10 / 3.21	3.36 / 2.91	3.71 / 3.64	3.16 / 3.24	3.02 / 3.17	3.50 / 3.46	3.23 / 3.08	3.40 / 3.01	3.07 / 3.07	3.21 / 3.22	3.20 / 2.99	3.14 / 3.17	3.27[c] / 3.14
Need more women doctors (1–5)	3.77 / 3.53	4.64[b] / 4.53[b]	3.92 / 3.79	4.29 / 3.98	3.96 / 3.79	4.12 / 3.74	4.06 / 3.98	4.07 / 3.71	4.10 / 3.90	3.98 / 3.81	4.09 / 4.00	3.88 / 3.79	3.96 / 3.71	4.19 / 3.52	4.01 / 3.79	4.03 / 3.90	3.93 / 3.66	4.08 / 3.97
Bias toward women patients (1–5)	2.89 / 2.85	3.46[b] / 3.86[b]	3.03 / 3.08	3.18 / 3.43	2.99 / 3.06	3.12 / 3.28	3.29 / 3.18	3.36 / 3.61	2.95 / 3.16	2.92 / 2.94	2.98 / 3.16	3.18 / 3.26	3.15 / 3.18	2.94 / 3.04	2.99 / 3.10	3.20[c] / 3.18	2.96 / 3.03	3.15[b] / 3.22
Number of cases	207	72	247	24	208	39	23	7	36	85	23	64	48	21	213	60	160	119

[a] For readability the interval variables, age and father's education, were each grouped into two categories. Age has been divided into 23 or less at the beginning of school and 24 or more at the onset of school. Father's education has been divided into college degree or less and more than a college degree. The tests of significance for the correlations of age and father's education with professional values and expectations were computed on the ungrouped data. The grouped data represent a rough approximation of the age and father's education effects.

[b] p < .01.

[c] p < .05.

TABLE 6.6

Standardized and Unstandardized Regression Coefficients for a Model of Professional Orientation Change concerning the Treatment of Women Physicians and Patients (with R^2 and constant for each equation)

Freshman-Year Professional Orientations and Explanatory Variables	Senior-Year Professional Orientations			
	Standardized Coefficients		Unstandardized Coefficients	
Bias toward Women Doctors				
Bias toward women doctors	.259[a]	.187[a]	.294[a]	.212[a]
Patients treated badly		.172[a]		.273[a]
Support women's movement		.195[a]		.245[a]
R^2	.067	.141		
Constant			2.037	.814
Specialty Choice Pressure				
Specialty choice pressure	.297[a]	.207[a]	.384[a]	.268[a]
Sex[c]	.238[a]	.154[b]	.307[a]	.407[b]
Race[c]	.237[a]	.136[b]	.625[a]	.552[b]
Urban background	.117[b]	-.114[b]	.477[c]	-.086[b]
Father's education	-.091	.084	-.068	.026
School[d]				
Duke		-.159[b]		-.392[b]
University of North Carolina		-.291[a]		-.679[a]
Patients treated badly		.269[a]		.474[a]
Support women's movement		.099		.138
Student treated badly		-.083		-.149
Active in liberal organizations		.044		.060
R^2	.088	.286		
Constant	1.929		1.783	.944

(continued)

TABLE 6.6 (continued)

Freshman-Year Professional Orientations and Explanatory Variables	Senior-Year Professional Orientations					
	Standardized Coefficients			Unstandardized Coefficients		
Need More Women Doctors						
Need more women doctors	.644[a]	.563[a]	.430[a]	.718[a]	.628[a]	.479[a]
Sex		.194[a]	.089		.453[a]	.207
Urban background		-.070	-.104[b]		-.046	-.069[b]
School						
Duke			.134[a]			.294[a]
University of North Carolina			.118[b]			.244[b]
Support women's movement			.375[a]			.464[a]
R²	.414	.451	.578			
Constant	.922	1.317	.603			
Bias toward Women Patients						
Bias toward women patients	.486[a]	.367[a]	.212[a]	.646[a]	.488[a]	.282[a]
Sex		.337[a]	.227[a]		.729[a]	.489[a]
Patients treated badly			.243[a]			.351[a]
Support women's movement			.274[a]			.314[a]
Student treated badly			.074			.108
Disagree with faculty			.077			.117
R²	.237	.336	.508			
Constant	1.149	1.441	-.387			

[a] p ≤ .01.
[b] p ≤ .05.
[c] Sex and race are coded so that males and whites equal zero and females and blacks equal one. All other variables are coded so that a high score indicates high on the variable as labeled.
[d] School has been recoded into three dummy variables. The omitted variable is Bowman Gray, which has regression coefficient equal to zero.

more, this table indicates that during training women become even more concerned than men with specialty choice pressure on women physicians (for example, pressure to choose pediatrics and to stay out of surgery), the need for more women physicians, and the prejudicial treatment of women patients. As another minority in medicine, blacks tended to begin and leave medical school more aware than whites of some of the problems faced by women in medicine, although these race differences were not for the most part statistically significant. Blacks, however, leave school significantly more conscious of specialty choice pressure on women physicians, although there was no race difference on this variable initially. Thus minority status—either being female or black—tends to promote more knowledge and support of women's issues. Other background characteristics of students did not seem particularly important in accounting for changes on women's issues.

When beginning medical school, there were no significant school differences among students on issues concerning the treatment of women physicians and patients (after controlling on background variables). Compared with other students, those at Bowman Gray (the omitted school category in Table 6.6) finished school less concerned with increasing the number of women physicians but more aware of specialty choice pressure on women in medicine. These school socialization effects appear somewhat contradictory at first glance. Bowman Gray is a more conservative institution than either the University of North Carolina or Duke, so it is not surprising that students there became even less supportive than others of increasing the number of women physicians. Bowman Gray students' greater concern with specialty choice pressure on women physicians was, however, contrary to expectation. Since Duke and the University of North Carolina appeared to be more liberal institutions, it might be that those students' decreased concerns with specialty choice pressure reflected better conditions for women at those schools. In fact, when women students at all schools were asked how stressful being a minority student had been since entering school, females at Bowman Gray were more likely to complain of stress (61 percent) than those at Duke (18 percent) or the University of North Carolina (38 percent).*

Finally, what seemed to explain most of the change on women's issues was whether students felt that patients were treated badly by faculty and attending physicians at their school, including how well

---

*These percentages are based on 18, 27, and 26 females who responded with at least "moderate stress" at Bowman Gray, Duke, and the University of North Carolina, respectively.

patients' social and psychological needs were met; and how familiar students were with the literature of the women's health movement and how much they supported the goals of that movement. Those who felt that patients were treated poorly and those who were supportive of the women's movement became even more concerned with the prejudicial treatment of women physicians and patients (see Table 6.6). Thus, rejecting the patient-care role models of the faculty and accepting an alternative ideology appeared to promote more critical views of the way women in medicine were treated. Most of the change on women's issues that was explained by school experiences was accounted for by students' views toward the treatment of patients and toward the women's movement. These explanatory variables were especially good at predicting how students' views changed concerning discrimination toward women patients. Thus, those students most likely to become skeptical of the claim that women patients experience discrimination were those who rejected the women's movement and accepted how their faculty treated patients.

PHYSICIAN MALDISTRIBUTION

From first to last year in medical school, students as a whole became less committed to choosing specialties and geographic areas that need physicians. Table 6.8 shows the background characteristics and school experiences that help explain some of this trend away from patient-need practices. This tendency away from needy areas probably reflects personal considerations as well as faculty bias against primary-care, rural, and inner-city practices.

Table 6.7 shows that females and males began medical school about equally committed to rural practice; however, females were slightly more likely to lose interest in such practices. Students' sex, however, did not predict any other changes in practice plans. Furthermore, race had a small role in explaining differential practice plans over time. Blacks began medical school much more committed than whites to inner-city ghetto practices and were more likely to remain interested in such practices during their training.

The type of background (for example, rural or urban) in which a student grew up seemed to have relevance for his or her commitment to patient need. Consistent with previous research,[3] Table 6.7 demonstrates that students from a rural background were somewhat more likely to begin medical school expecting to practice in a rural area and were considerably less likely to lose interest in rural practice

TABLE 6.7

Means on Freshman and Senior Professional Orientations concerning Physician Maldistribution by Students' Background Characteristics

Freshman/Senior Year (range of values)

Professional Orientations	Sex Male	Sex Female	Race White	Race Black	Religion Protestant	Religion Catholic	Religion Jewish	Religion None	Background Rural	Background Small Town	Background Suburb, Medium City	Background Medium City	Background Suburb, Large City	Background Large City	Age[a] (freshman year) 23 or Less	Age[a] (freshman year) 24 or More	Father's Education[a] College or Less	Father's Education[a] More than College
Primary-care plans (1–5)	3.83 / 3.22	3.92 / 3.32	3.85 / 3.21	3.77 / 3.56	3.97 / 3.41	3.53 / 2.78	3.51 / 2.74	3.07[b] / 2.57[c]	4.35 / 3.99	3.88 / 3.33	4.02 / 3.37	3.70 / 2.86	3.63 / 3.06	3.79[c] / 3.02[b]	3.80 / 3.22	4.03 / 3.32	3.96 / 3.47	3.72[c] / 2.95[b]
Rural practice plans (1–4)	2.58 / 2.13	2.49 / 1.88[c]	2.53 / 2.06	2.54 / 2.00	2.58 / 2.12	2.51 / 1.95	2.39 / 1.74	2.29 / 1.71	3.14 / 2.92	2.61 / 1.99	2.39 / 1.74	2.42 / 1.95	2.44 / 1.90	2.10[b] / 1.90[b]	2.50 / 2.06	2.68 / 2.03	2.71 / 2.23	2.34[b] / 1.84[b]
Inner-city practice plans (1–4)	1.89 / 1.46	2.18[b] / 1.72[b]	1.87 / 1.45	2.88[b] / 2.42[b]	1.95 / 1.48	2.05 / 1.68	1.96 / 1.70	2.14 / 1.57	1.92 / 1.42	1.89 / 1.39	1.74 / 1.91	2.05 / 1.66	1.88 / 1.40	2.48[c] / 1.75[c]	1.98 / 1.55	1.90 / 1.47	2.02 / 1.54	1.89[c] / 1.51
Committed to patient need (1–5)	3.68 / 3.15	3.39[c] / 3.01	3.55 / 3.05	4.06[c] / 3.53	3.66 / 3.22	3.52 / 2.85	3.30 / 2.23	3.23 / 2.36[c]	4.23 / 3.82	3.51 / 3.12	3.37 / 2.67	3.43 / 2.97	3.66 / 2.90	3.59[b] / 3.24[b]	3.58 / 3.09	3.67 / 3.16	3.70 / 3.28	3.48[c] / 2.89[b]
Number of cases[d]	207	72	247	24	208	39	23	7	36	85	23	64	48	21	213	60	160	119

[a] For readability the interval variables, age and father's education, were each grouped into two categories. Age has been divided into 23 or less at the beginning of school and 24 or more at the onset of school. Father's education has been divided into college degree or less and more than a college degree. The tests of significance for the correlations of age and father's education with professional values and expectations were computed on the ungrouped data. The grouped data represent a rough approximation of the age and father's education effects.

[b] p < .01.

[c] p < .05.

[d] Calculations are based on the number of cases shown except for the single-item measures (rural practice plans and inner-city practice plans) computed on slightly fewer cases.

131

TABLE 6.8

Standardized and Unstandardized Regression Coefficients for a Model of Professional Orientation Change concerning Physician Maldistribution
(with R^2 and constant for each equation)

Freshman-Year Professional Orientations and Explanatory Variables	Senior-Year Professional Orientations			
	Standardized Coefficients		Unstandardized Coefficients	
	Primary-Care Plans		Primary-Care Plans	

Primary-Care Plans

Variable	Standardized		Unstandardized	
Primary-care plans	.406[a]	.355[a]	.546[a]	.478[a]
School[c]				
Duke	-.190[a]		-.617[a]	
University of North Carolina	.079		.242	
Disagree with faculty	.130[b]		.318[b]	
Encourage primary care	-.259[a]	.265	-.382[a]	
R^2	.165			
Constant			1.144	1.809

Rural Practice Plans

Variable	Standardized		Unstandardized	
Rural practice plans	.485[a]	.271[a]	.490[a]	.274[a]
Sex[d]	-.110[b]	-.127[a]	-.256[b]	-.296[a]
Race[d]	-.053	-.088[b]	-.189	-.313[b]
Background[b]				
Rural	.256[a]	.187[a]	.774[a]	.565[a]
Small town	.022	-.006	.048	-.013
Suburb, medium city	-.033	-.067	-.121	-.248
Medium city	.045	.076	.108	.183
Large city	.057	.041	.219	.157
Age	-.061	-.095[b]	-.033	-.051[b]
School debts		.108[b]		.010[b]
Primary-care plans (senior)		.489[a]		.327[a]
R^2	.235	.306	.518	.813
Constant			1.731	1.516

Inner-City Practice Plans

	(1)	(2)	(3)	(4)	(5)	(6)
Inner-city practice plans	.466[a]	.399[a]	.360[a]	.474[a]	.406[a]	.366[a]
Race		.211[a]	.222[a]		.594[a]	.624[a]
Background						
Rural		-.037	-.080		-.087	-.191
Small town		-.033	-.049		-.057	-.085
Suburb, medium city		.199[a]	.188[a]		.575[a]	.543[a]
Medium city		.056	.050		.107	.094
Large city		.005	.010		.015	.030
Experience school difficulty			.120[b]			.105[b]
Primary-care plans (senior)			.110[b]			.058[b]
R^2	.218	.299	.327			
Constant				.598	.634	.224

Committed to Patient Need

	(1)	(2)	(3)	(4)	(5)	(6)
Committed to patient need	.549[a]	.549[a]	.317[a]	.655[a]	.654[a]	.378[a]
Age		-.024	-.127[a]		-.016	-.084[a]
Children[d]			.114[b]			.419[b]
School						
Duke			.020			.054
University of North Carolina			.113[b]			.286[b]
Academic medicine plans (senior)			-.161[a]			-.232[a]
Primary-care plans (senior)			-.407[a]			.335[a]
View career negatively			-.122[a]			-.139[a]
Grades in school			-.085			-.112
Experience school difficulty			.082			.112
R^2	.302	.302	.581			
Constant				.752	1.162	3.899

[a] $p \leq .01$.

[b] $p \leq .05$.

[c] School and background were recoded into dummy variables. The omitted variable of the three school variables is Bowman Gray. The omitted variable of the six background variables is "suburb of a large city." The rural/urban background variable was recoded into dummy variables because it was found to be nonlinearly related to some of the distribution issues. The regression coefficients for both omitted categories are equal to zero.

[d] Sex, race, and children are coded so that males, whites, and having no children equal zero and females, blacks, and having children equal one. All other variables are coded so that a high score indicates high on the variable as labeled.

through training.* Thus, medical school admission committees have wisely realized that one way to increase the proportion of physicians in patient-need areas has been to select students from these locations. Table 6.7 also shows that students from the suburbs of a medium city tended to gain interest in inner-city practice, whereas students from other types of backgrounds tended to lose interest in such practices. This seems ironic because those from the suburbs of a medium city were least likely to choose inner-city practice during freshman year. In summary, those from large cities, medium cities, and especially the suburbs of medium cities end up the most interested in inner-city ghetto practice. This is consistent with the theory that people tend to live in areas similar to the ones in which they grew up. In this case, people from cities are more likely than others to choose such city practice locations as ghettos.

Lower class students (as indicated in Table 6.7 by father's education) began and finished medical school with a greater commitment to such needed practices as primary-care and rural medicine.† Thus, recruiting working-class students into medical school may be one way to improve physician specialty and geographic distribution.

Even controlling on students' social background characteristics, freshmen at Duke were less oriented to primary-care medicine than freshmen at the other two schools. Thus students select Duke and are admitted into that institution in part because of their greater interest in research and specialty medicine. Duke has a reputation for training researchers and teachers as opposed to primary-care clinicians because they have a combined degree program (M.D. and Ph.D.) for those interested in academic medicine. In fact, when seniors were asked, "To what extent do faculty and housestaff at your school encourage students to choose primary-care practice," 18 percent of the Duke students indicated encouragement as compared with 59 percent and 63 percent of those at the University of North Carolina and Bowman Gray, respectively. Thus, it is not surprising that Duke students were slightly less likely than others to maintain their plans to practice

---

*Although freshmen from rural areas were also more likely to plan primary-care careers, this was partially due to differences on other background attributes.

†The initial difference between the social classes on inner-city practice plans was largely accounted for by blacks' greater commitment to inner-city medicine. Because blacks tend to be from lower socioeconomic-status families, this socioeconomic-status difference was mainly a reflection of a race difference.

primary-care medicine as they went through training (see Table 6. 8). On the other hand, students at all schools were equally likely to lose interest in rural practice from first to last year in medical school.

The author previously noted that all schools were less encouraging of primary-care than specialty medicine. The following statement from a student at the University of North Carolina indicates this specialization bias.

> I met a few people in my clinical years who tried to say
> to me that it's okay, that you could do general medicine
> and you could do it adequately, but they were only a few.
> Most of the people at a place like this, the attendings
> you work with, are specialists and they try to get across
> to you either consciously or subconsciously the idea that
> you've got to go at it the way they did, which is to spe-
> cialize. You had to know all the esoterica in order to
> practice medicine.

Table 6. 8 shows that students who disagreed with the faculty and attending physicians' political views were somewhat less likely to lose their commitment to primary-care medicine. Staying in primary care was facilitated by some degree of rebelliousness or at least rejection of dominant norms. Likewise, primary-care plans were somewhat inhibited by accepting faculty role models. More striking, however, is the finding that those who felt their school discouraged primary-care medicine were the ones most likely to stay in that field. (Note the negative sign on the regression coefficient in Table 6. 8 under primary-care plans [-.259]). At first glance, one would assume that those who felt discouragement for primary care would be the ones to leave it. It seems that sensitivity to whether primary care was encouraged or discouraged was much stronger among those who selected these fields. Thus, those who remained in primary-care fields recognized and felt more acutely the negative attitudes that they encountered due to this choice. Staying in primary care required rejecting the dominant professional views of the specialists who compose the medical school faculty, such as attitudes that equate primary care with incompetence.

Seniors who were interested in primary-care medicine were also less likely to change their plans away from practices in rural and inner-city areas and by definition stayed more committed to choosing patient-need practices (see Table 6. 8). These findings are consistent with the evidence that primary-care medicine plans are highly positively correlated with rural practice and slightly positively correlated with inner-city practice. Choosing primary-care medicine was a much better predictor of who will remain interested in rural practices than who will continue to plan inner-city practices.

As with interest in volunteer work and helping people, experiencing school difficulty in terms of time pressures slightly maintained commitment to inner-city ghetto practice (see Table 6.8). Contrary to expectation, feeling that school was difficult and involved sacrifices due to the long hours did not make students less altruistic in their motivations or career plans. In fact, those who felt these time pressures were slightly more likely to maintain their plans to help people through volunteer work and inner-city practice. Perhaps those who felt the time constraints most were the students most involved with volunteer and service activities before starting medical school. Experiencing time constraints and working hard may more aptly describe the type of student who did service work prior to school and who continues to do such work rather than serve as a reason for maintaining interest in such altruistic pursuits. Thus, some students may feel more time pressures because they are more altruistic and service oriented.

Contrary to expectation, having large school debts did not lead to more conservative and less service-oriented values and career priorities. For the most part, having school debts was unimportant in predicting change on professional values and expectations. Those with large debts, however, were slightly less inclined to lose interest in rural practice (see Table 6.8). From an economic point of view this does not make much sense, because rural physicians have traditionally made less money than urban physicians. But federally and state funded loan-forgiveness programs reduce the debts of students with such loans if they practice in needy areas.[4] Thus, perhaps the reason that students with high debts remained slightly more committed to rural practice was due to the economic incentives of loan-forgiveness programs. Furthermore, those with high debts were also more likely to be from less economically privileged homes. Since rural practice is more popular with lower class students, perhaps debts are a proxy for family's economic standing.

Viewing one's career and medical education negatively, unlike experiencing difficulty and time constraints in school, did seem to adversely affect students' altruistic motivations. Students who left medical school with negative feelings about their education and who questioned if they had chosen the right profession were less likely to maintain a commitment to patient need and, as shown before, less likely to remain concerned with helping people. Thus simply working hard and feeling the time pressures and constraints of medical school does not lead to less altruism. If training, however, results in disliking medical school and the profession, then this rejection is reflected in the negation of other goals, such as the humanitarian ones.

Other than the factors already mentioned, many considera-
ations affect students' specialization and location plans. Medical
training encourages dependence on modern hospital technology and
interest in rare as opposed to chronic and common illnesses, training that is not compatible with rural and primary-care practice.
Personal considerations, like wanting to work fewer and more regular
hours and not wanting to be isolated from colleagues, also tend to
divert students away from patient-need practices. Coupled with personal considerations, professional socialization seems to further
discourage students from choosing the types of practices that would
help alleviate some health-care deficiencies.

FURTHER EXPLANATIONS OF CHANGE
AND CONCLUSIONS

In this chapter, the author has explored some of the reasons
underlying the changes in professional values and expectations that
have occurred in medical school. By and large, rejecting medical
school role models (that is, rejecting physicians' views toward political issues and the way they treat patients) and advocating such alternative ideologies as those connected with the women's movement
helped students resist growing conservatism on political, economic,
and women's issues in medicine. Activity in minority and liberal organizations for the most part did not prevent growing conservatism.
Rejecting the faculty's and attending physicians' political views (the
values held by specialists) also helped to slow up the trend toward
specialization. Furthermore, supporting the women's movement
and rejecting the medical faculty's political ideology contributed to
maintaining more egalitarian views toward the treatment of patients.

We are then left wondering why some students were able to go
through four years of medical training and continue to reject most
faculty role models and to hold alternative values, whereas others
succumbed more totally to the socialization process. Unfortunately,
the present analysis can give us no more insight into this issue, since
it has focused primarily on school experiences rather than on personality and on other life experiences that might contribute to change.
Thus, the author has not attempted to explore all possible causes of
professional orientation change, only those related to professional
socialization.

The main conclusion from the analysis in this chapter is that
in order to sustain liberal and patient-oriented perspectives and plans,
it helps if students reject some of the values consciously or unconsciously taught in medical school as well as adopt alternative liberal

ideologies. In talking about the conservative trend in medical school one male student at Bowman Gray said the following:

> You are essentially being trained by conservative people here at the institution. You might be a liberal type person to start, but as you get into the system and become pounded by conservatism. . .the general conservatism of the older faculty, you learn to quit fighting the system as much and become more docile and more established.

Those who do not quit fighting the system may remain more liberal, egalitarian, and patient oriented in their views and career plans.

It is unclear whether rejecting faculty views and being familiar with the women's movement lead to more liberal professional values or whether more liberal professional views lead to rejecting the faculty and being receptive to women's causes. These causal priorities are difficult to pin down because the data do not trace the socialization experience during four years of medical school. The important issue, however, is not whether fighting the system leads to liberalism or vice versa, but that rejecting faculty views and supporting women's causes seem related to maintaining values and expectations that facilitate what has been defined here as good health care.

The author has presented evidence that medical school is a conservative environment that tends to reinforce conservative values on political and economic issues in medicine. Furthermore, it tends to promote careers that do not meet critical health needs. Other factors contributing to these changes over time may be the conservative trend nationally, aging, and maturing. It is apparent that this country is getting more conservative politically since the era of the 1960s and early 1970s. One could argue that perhaps the change from 1975 to 1978 in most medical students' views toward political and economic issues in medicine was due to a change in their political liberalism over time. This hypothesis was tested, and change in general political outlook (becoming more conservative) accounted only somewhat for becoming more protective of the profession's right to control health care. Change in general political outlook did not explain changes on any other professional value or expectation. Thus, the conservative trend nationally did not appear to explain decreasing liberalism on most professional orientations.

There is something to be said for the possible conservative effects of aging and maturing, that is, being better informed and more realistic about what can and cannot be changed and getting closer to joining the professional ranks of a high-status position in society.

The effects of becoming older are explained by the following male respondents.

> Whereas when you started out you may be more lib-
> eral and think a lot of changes should be made so-
> cially. . .when you get down to it, its not going to
> be done so you may as well not consider it. . . .
> You can't make a poor family not poor. You can't
> make a dumb, illiterate family smart enough to
> take care of themselves on a complex problem.

> I think medical school is not going to make you more
> liberal and most of my friends I think feel the same
> way because just in your thinking a physician oc-
> cupies a reasonably status oriented position in so-
> ciety. Anybody with that position, if anything, is
> going to want to preserve the status quo. . . . Now
> we have to start thinking about our career, what kind
> of life-style do we want when we get out of school.

Although there are many factors not all related to school experiences that affected students' professional values and expectations,
it appeared that students' liberal values and commitment to patient-
need practices have been somewhat undermined by medical training,
a training led by specialists and conservatively oriented professors.
If future doctors are going to be concerned with many of our present
health-care problems, then medical schools will have to reexamine
the implicit and explicit values and career biases taught in medical
school.

In addition to showing which school experiences have contributed
to professional orientation change, this chapter has explored the role
that student's background characteristics have played in predicting
initial and senior-year orientations. It seems that such minority
student statuses as being black, working class, and from a rural
area contributed to beginning and finishing school with a greater commitment to patient-need practices. Being female and/or black also
promoted a more liberal outlook on a variety of issues. Thus, the
medical profession and the practice of medicine could be improved
if medical schools adopt affirmative action programs to recruit students from minority statuses, that is, those groups underrepresented
in medicine today. In the next chapter, the professional orientations
of men and women are compared during their first and last years of
school.

NOTES

1. Lee J. Cronbach and Lita Furby, "Can We Measure Change—or Should We?" Psychological Bulletin 69 (1970): 68-80.

2. For a discussion of regressed change analysis, see ibid.

3. Mark Taylor, William Dickman, and Robert Kane, "Medical Students' Attitudes toward Rural Practice," Journal of Medical Education 48 (October 1973): 885-95.

4. Charles E. Lewis, Rashi Fein, and David Mechanic, A Right to Health: The Problem of Access to Primary Medical Care (New York: John Wiley & Sons, 1976), pp. 47-60.

7

COMPARING MEN AND WOMEN

Because of the previous scarcity of women in medicine, research on medical students until recently has neglected comparisons of the professional orientations of men and women. Furthermore, few studies have examined how the socialization process in medical school might differ for the sexes. Although some recent studies have examined gender differences on values and career choices,[1] existing research on women in medicine has focused primarily on the problems women face in a male profession and in balancing career and family commitments. Thus, this chapter presents one of the main and unique themes of this book, that is, the relationship over time between students' gender and professional values and expectations. Two main questions are addressed: Do males and females differ in their professional orientations upon entrance to medical school? Do the professional orientation differences between males and females persist until senior year, or does professional socialization tend to have a homogenizing effect? The issues of why the sexes differ upon entrance to school and why they may change differently over time will be discussed in Chapter 8.

As expected, female medical students do in fact enter school with more liberal and humanitarian values than their male peers. These initial gender differences in professional orientations were expected to at least persist through medical training. The emergence of some new sex differences in professional orientations and the widening of some initial ones were further anticipated because of such factors as the isolation and discrimination experienced by women in a male profession and the formation of alternative women's reference groups. Thus, a less orderly socialization of women in medical school was expected to result in less conformity to professional values for women when compared with men.

Gender comparisons in professional orientations should suggest ways that the recent increase in the proportion of women in medical school may affect the practice and profession of medicine. If women hold different values and choose different types of medical careers than men, the influx of women in medicine may have implications for health-care delivery and quality.

SEX DIFFERENCES IN PROFESSIONAL
ORIENTATIONS OVER TIME

Upon entrance to medical school, women are more oriented than men to humanizing doctor/patient interactions, supporting political and economic change in medicine, being aware of the problems facing women physicians and patients, and expecting an inner-city ghetto practice. Because students' sex was essentially unrelated to most other social background characteristics (for example, race and social class), the initial statistically significant sex differences in professional orientations were virtually unchanged when controlling on background variables. In other words, the differences between first-year men and women on professional orientations were not explained by sex differences on background characteristics.* In addition, the relationship between sex and professional orientation for the most part did not vary across levels or categories of selected background variables. For example, sex differences on professional orientations were approximately the same at all schools, so that the three institutions were combined in the data analysis with no loss of information.†

———————————

*The social background characteristics measured in freshman year that were examined for their possible confounding of the initial relationship between sex and professional orientations are listed in Chapter 3 under the heading "Social Background Attributes." All background variables have been tested for nonlinearity and all were found to be linearly related to the professional orientation measures.

†The few statistically significant interactions between sex and selected background measures (race, medical school, social class, marital status, and religion) on the professional orientations can be dismissed as random events, since at the .05 level of significance we would expect 5 significant interactions out of 100 because of chance alone. Although sex differences in orientation were somewhat greater at some schools than others, these interactions were not significant owing to the small number of women at each of the institutions.

Tables 7.1, 7.2, 7.3, and 7.6 present the means, standard deviations, and percentage distributions on professional orientation measures for men and women during their freshman and senior years, the correlation of each measure from time 1 to time 2 computed separately for men and women, and the T-test for dependent samples indicating significant differences in the means over time for each sex.* The correlation coefficients reported in these tables indicate to what extent individuals in each sex category are consistent in their scores on variables from freshman to senior year. The T-tests show whether women or men as a whole have changed over time. The discussion comparing men and women from first to last year on the professional orientations will be organized around the four health-care problem areas.

Physicians' Relationships with Patients

As noted previously, medical schools and medical professionals have been criticized for their lack of attention to the problems of humanizing and equalizing doctor/patient interactions. Recently, there has been speculation that women will add a touch of humanity to medicine resulting from the greater nurturance and empathy associated with traditional female socialization.

Table 7.1 shows that, contrary to expectation, male and female students in their first year did not differ significantly on attitudes concerning the importance of providing health information to patients and of patients being critical of physicians' judgments (values concerning egalitarian patient care). Later, however, we see that females do tend to hold more humanitarian patient-care views during the first year. The author had expected females to support more egalitarian doctor/patient relationships because traditional sex role socialization emphasizes greater nurturance and less dominance in relating to other people. Personality measures indicating nurturance

---

*The results of a one-tailed T-test for differences between males and females on each orientation are indicated next to the male means. A one-tailed (as opposed to a two-tailed) T-test was used because in most cases hypotheses were directional. In addition, owing to slight variations in the means when computed on the subset of the population that answered both questionnaires (279) as compared with computations based on all those who answered the first questionnaire (326), the one-tailed T-test results more closely parallel the original findings on 326 cases.

TABLE 7.1

Means, Standard Deviations, and Percentage Distributions on Measures concerning the Doctor/Patient Relationship for Males and Females during Their Freshman and Senior Years in Medical School, 1975 and 1978 (with correlation coefficients between measures across time and T-tests for dependent samples)

| | Freshman Year, 1975 | | | | | Senior Year, 1978 | | | | | | |
| | Index Score[a] | | Percentage in Each Category | | | Index Score | | Percentage in Each Category | | | | |
Variable	Mean	Standard Deviation	Disagree	Neutral	Agree	Mean	Standard Deviation	Disagree	Neutral	Agree	T-Test	r
Important to provide health information to patients												
Male	3.25	0.79	23.2	35.7	41.1	3.24[b]	0.78	24.2	27.1	48.8	0.19	.42
Female	3.34	0.77	20.8	37.5	41.7	3.48	0.73	11.1	33.3	55.6	1.46	.42
Patients should not have absolute confidence in physicians' judgments												
Male	2.78	1.09	46.4	20.3	33.3	3.29[b]	1.02	27.1	25.6	47.3	6.76[d]	.46
Female	2.93	1.05	45.8	15.3	38.9	3.55	0.95	22.2	15.3	62.5	4.54[d]	.33
Social and psychological factors, including empathy, are important in health care												
Male	4.25[c]	0.54	—	9.2	90.8	4.27[c]	0.59	0.5	11.1	88.4	0.38	.36
Female	4.54	0.51	—	4.2	95.8	4.50	0.49	0.0	5.6	94.4	0.45	.25
Chose medicine in order to help people (helping people is an important part of medical career)[a]												
Male	3.31[b]	0.61	10.6	—	89.4	3.11	0.62	19.8	—	80.2	4.35[d]	.44
Female	3.45	0.47	5.6	—	94.4	3.19	0.65	19.4	—	80.6	3.58[d]	.41

r = correlation coefficient

[a] All variables are indexes composed of two or more questionnaire items calculated on 207 males and 72 females. The range of possible values is one to five for all measures except choosing medicine in order to help people, which ranges from one to four. On this variable, the approximate wording on the 1978 questionnaire is shown in parentheses. On indexes ranging from one to five, scores of 1.0 to 2.50 are labeled "disagree," scores of 2.51 to 3.49 are labeled "neutral," and scores of 3.50 to 5.0 are labeled "agree." On the measure coded from one to four, scores of 1.0 to 2.50 are labeled "disagree," and scores of 2.51 to 4.0 are labeled "agree."

[b] Indicates a p < .05 of a significant difference between the male and female means using a one-tailed T-test.

[c] Indicates a p < .01 of a significant difference between the male and female means using a one-tailed T-test.

[d] Indicates T-tests have a p < .01 of a significant difference in orientation from freshman to senior year using a two-tailed T-test.

and dominance, however, were uncorrelated with these two values concerning egalitarian doctor/patient relationships. As shown in Table 6.1, social class (having an educated father) was a better predictor than sex of these egalitarian attitudes, at least upon entrance to medical school.

Although as freshmen the sexes did not significantly differ on the importance they attached to providing health information to patients and to patients being critical of physicians' judgments, in the senior year women were somewhat more committed than men to both of these values aimed at involving patients in health-care decisions. Because males as a group have placed the same importance over time on providing health information to patients and females have become slightly more concerned with this issue, a significant sex difference emerged during senior year (24.2 percent of the males disagreed with this issue compared with 11.1 percent of the females). This finding is consistent with a recent study of physicians suggesting that women are more open and honest with dying patients than are men. [2] Although both sexes appear to more realistically appraise physicians' limitations in the senior year, females became slightly more in favor of patients being critical of physicians' judgments (62.5 percent) than the males (47.3 percent). Sex differences in the senior year on values concerning the giving of health information to patients and patients being critical of physicians were the result of women both starting out and becoming slightly more egalitarian on these issues than men.

Although most freshmen emphasized the importance of humanizing doctor/patient relationships, women placed somewhat more importance than men on the need to establish rapport with patients and to understand patients' social and psychological problems. In addition, Table 7.1 shows that upon entrance to medical school women tended to express their desire to help people (94.4 percent) slightly more than the men expressed this concern (89.4 percent). These findings are consistent with some other studies of physicians, medical school applicants, and medical students indicating that women are more nurturant than men and are more likely to value close patient relationships. [3]

Because neither males nor females changed significantly over time in the importance they attached to social and psychological factors in health care, females have remained more committed to these ideals. Although initially females were more likely to choose medicine in order to help people, the sex difference on this humanitarian value did not persist through senior year. Over time, both males and females tended to view helping people as slightly less integral to their careers.

Both sexes experienced some individual fluctuation on all professional values concerning the doctor/patient relationship from freshman to senior year, although females tended to fluctuate slightly more than males (as shown in the lower correlations across time for women). Overall, however, females left medical school with more humanitarian and egalitarian patient-care values than men. By and large, professional socialization did not seem to have a detrimental effect on the patient-care values of most students, because males and especially females tended to become more sensitive to issues of patient involvement in health-care decisions. The socialization process appeared to have a slightly different effect on males and females, although the effects on both sexes were fairly small in most cases.

In summary, women begin school with more humanitarian patient-care values but do not differ from men on egalitarian issues of care. As they leave school, women hold both more humanitarian and egalitarian views.

Because women leave medical school more oriented to values that emphasize patient involvement in health-care decisions, in practice they may develop more egalitarian relationships with patients marked by better communication and rapport. The increase in the proportion of women in medicine may in fact add a needed touch of humanity to the practice of medicine.

Political and Economic Change in the Medical Profession

Controversial reforms calling for government intervention in health care, the elimination of profits made by health institutions, and the lowering of income made by physicians address major problems with the present health-care system. Compared with men, women were expected to begin medical school more strongly advocating and planning to work for such political and economic reforms in medicine. Table 7.2 shows that this expectation was for the most part substantiated.

Among freshmen, females tended to more strongly advocate political change in the medical profession including government intervention in health care. About 44 percent of the women favored a reduction in the profession's control over health through reforms like socialized medicine, and 28 percent supported a compulsory National Service Corps for physicians to serve in deprived areas (even without payment for medical education) compared with 29 percent and about 17 percent of the men, respectively. Furthermore, women began medical school advocating more radical changes, such as favoring the elimination of profits made by drug companies, insurance companies, and hospitals (54.2 percent) to a much greater extent than did the men (36.4 percent).

Women also tended to be less oriented to large income and status. Among freshmen, women were substantially more likely to support the lowering of physicians' income and status rewards (56.9 percent) compared with the men (30.0 percent). This finding is compatible with women's lower interest in high income and prestige, indicated by both the data in this study (15.3 percent compared with 24.6 percent for men) and previous research. [4]

Finally, among freshmen, women tended to plan to work for political and social change in medicine (37.5 percent) slightly more than the men (29.0 percent). Although women expected to do slightly more volunteer work than the men, these differences in volunteer plans were not statistically significant. Women did not differ as much from men on planning work that would lead to social and political change as they did on reformist values. Women, however, were consistently more liberal on political and economic change issues upon entrance to medical school.

Although both males and females became significantly more conservative over time on all issues concerning political and economic change in medicine, the large initial sex differences on these professional orientations persisted through senior year. Thus, medical school has a similar conservative effect on both men and women, but women end up supporting more liberal values because they started with more liberal views. Therefore, the differences between men and women remained fairly constant on almost all professional orientations concerning political and economic change. If the means for males and females on most political and economic change variables were plotted on a graph from freshman to senior year, the picture would show two nearly parallel downward slopes (down indicating greater conservatism).

Thus, despite growing conservatism, females were still more likely during the senior year to favor a reduction in the profession's control over health care (37.5 percent) and change in the profit system (34.7 percent) in contrast to the men (16.9 percent and 18.8 percent, respectively). Seniors became less supportive of a National Service Corps regardless of the remuneration involved, although more males rejected such a plan (47.3 percent) when compared with the females (31.9 percent). Furthermore, among seniors men were still more oriented to money so that more men rejected plans to lower physicians' financial and status rewards (51.2 percent), and more men considered income and status an important part of their careers (33.3 percent) compared with the women (23.6 percent and 19.4 percent, respectively). Although students overall became less likely to plan political and social change work in medicine, in the senior year women continued to expect such work (30.6 percent) more than the men (15.0 percent).

Contrary to all the findings just enumerated, in the senior year men planned slightly more volunteer work (about 12 percent of their

TABLE 7.2

Means, Standard Deviations, and Percentage Distributions on Measures concerning Political and Economic Change in the Medical Profession for Males and Females during Their Freshman and Senior Years in Medical School, 1975 and 1978 (with correlation coefficients between measures across time and T-tests for dependent samples)

| | Freshman Year, 1975 | | | | | Senior Year, 1978 | | | | | | |
| | Index Score[a] | | Percentage in Each Category | | | Index Score | | Percentage in Each Category | | | | |
Variable	Mean	Standard Deviation	Low	Middle	High	Mean	Standard Deviation	Low	Middle	High	T-Test	r
Profession's control over health should be reduced through government intervention and socialized medicine												
Male	2.88[c]	1.02	37.7	33.3	29.0	2.41[d]	0.96	57.5	25.6	16.9	7.43	.58
Female	3.19	1.01	27.8	27.8	44.4	2.90	1.04	37.5	25.0	37.5	2.84	.63
Favor a compulsory National Service Corps for physicians to serve in deprived areas												
Male	1.89[d]	0.66	27.5	55.9	16.7	1.68[c]	0.72	47.3	37.6	15.1	3.79	.34
Female	2.11	0.67	16.9	54.9	28.2	1.86	0.70	31.9	50.0	18.1	2.92	.43
The health-care system needs to be changed to that profits cannot be made												
Male	2.85[d]	1.21	49.0	14.6	36.4	2.28[d]	1.13	71.0	10.1	18.8	7.34	.53
Female	3.33	1.27	36.1	9.7	54.2	2.78	1.21	52.8	12.5	34.7	3.76	.49
Physicians' status and financial rewards need to be lowered												
Male	2.98[d]	0.83	35.3	34.8	30.0	2.67[d]	0.86	51.2	27.1	21.7	6.12	.64
Female	3.38	0.72	18.1	25.0	56.9	3.02	0.78	23.6	45.8	30.6	4.07	.51
High status and income were important in career selection												

(high status and income are important part of medical career)[a]

Male	1.99[d]	0.60	75.4	39.3	—	24.6	2.16[c]	0.59	66.7	—	33.3	4.68	.60
Female	1.80	0.55	84.7	32.4	—	15.3	1.98	0.56	80.6	—	19.4	2.64	.44
Expect to work for political and social change in medicine													
Male	2.12[c]	0.71	71.0	—	—	29.0	1.79[d]	0.68	85.0	—	15.0	6.84	.50
Female	2.31	0.81	62.5	—	—	37.5	2.06	0.82	69.4	—	30.6	3.28	.69
Percentage of time expect to do volunteer work													
Male	17.09	11.54	39.8	39.3	23.8	20.9	11.92[c]	8.40	66.3	23.8	9.9	7.61	.57
Female	18.74	11.60	35.3	32.4	27.1	32.4	9.91	6.17	71.4	27.1	1.4	5.84	.18

r = correlation coefficient

[a]Variables are indexes composed of two or more questionnaire items with the exception of favoring a National Service Corps, favoring a change in the health-care system, and planning volunteer work, which are single-item measures. All calculations are based on 207 cases for males and 72 cases for females as a result of missing data. The range of possible values is one to five on favoring government intervention, a change in the health-care system, and lower financial rewards for physicians. On these measures, scores of 1.0 to 2.50 are labeled "low," scores of 2.51 to 3.49 are labeled "middle," and scores of 3.50 to 5.0 are labeled "high." The range of possible values is one to four on the importance of high status and income and expecting to work for change. On these measures, scores of 1.0 to 2.50 are labeled "low," and scores of 2.51 to 4.0 are labeled "high." The approximate wording on the 1978 questionnaire for the importance of high income and status is shown in parentheses. The single item favoring a National Service Corps ranges from one to three, so that the three responses "no," "yes, only if medical education is paid," and "yes," are labeled "low," "middle," and "high," respectively. The percentage of time one plans volunteer work has a possible range of 0 to 100 percent, so that 0 to 10 percent is labeled "low," 11 to 20 percent is labeled "middle," and 21 percent and over is labeled "high."

[b]All T-tests have a $p \leq .01$ of a significant difference in orientation from freshman to senior year using a two-tailed T-test.

[c]Indicates a $p < .05$ of a significant difference between the male and female means using a one-tailed T-test.

[d]Indicates a $p < .01$ of a significant difference between the male and female means using a one-tailed T-test.

149

practice time) than women (about 10 percent of their practice time). All students became less likely to plan volunteer work; however, women decreased their volunteer plans more drastically. The low correlation between the time 1 and time 2 volunteer work measures for women indicates great individual fluctuation.

When students were asked in the senior year, "On the average, how many hours a week do you want to work when you finish your medical training?" males wanted to work significantly more hours (52.4 hours) than females (47.8 hours). But when questioned about the hours they expected to work, the sexes did not significantly differ (61.2 hours for men and 62.9 hours for women). In the senior year, therefore, males and especially females planned to work on the average more than they wanted. It seems plausible that some volunteer work expectations were dropped, especially among women, because students already were expecting to work more than they preferred. In addition, during freshman year the men were fairly realistic about the amount of time they expected to work (men expected to work an average of 61.5 hours a week which was similar to their senior-year estimates); however, in their freshman year women expected to work far fewer hours (56.2 hours) than they did as seniors. Women's realizations of the larger work load may have also contributed to their declining interest in volunteer work. In addition, the added time pressures on women to raise a family and manage a career probably make volunteer work a more optional, although valued, goal. The issue of why women change their volunteer plans more than men will be discussed further in Chapter 8.

The fairly high correlation coefficients between most of the time one and time two indexes concerning political and economic change for both males and females indicate a fairly uniform group change with little individual attitudinal fluctuation. Although medical school appears to have a conservative impact on most students, professional socialization has not obliterated sex differences on political and economic change values. Females have continued to espouse more liberal stances on political and economic issues, although males have started to plan more time doing volunteer work. Originally the author proposed that such factors as the isolation of women in medical school, the lack of female role models, and the formation of women's groups with alternative ideologies would prevent medical school from having a conservative influence on women. For the most part, on issues concerning political and economic change in medicine, this appeared not to be the case. Thus socialization seemed to have a similar influence on both sexes; medical student status (or anticipated physician status) was apparently more important than gender in determining much of the attitudinal change. Socialization, however, was not a great leveler of attitudinal variation, because the conservative influence of medical training was not strong enough to wipe out or reduce initial sex differences. In other words, medical school does not eliminate the baseline sex differences, despite its conservative effect.

Assuming that senior-year values indicate something about subsequent behavior, the author expects that by and large women will have a liberalizing effect on the profession. Women's greater enthusiasm for reforms like socialized medicine and lower physician income may translate in practice into charging lower fees than men and being more responsive to public health needs. One recent study of physicians found that females did, in fact, receive lower fees than males for the same procedures.[5] Because doctors set their own fee schedules, it would seem that women's lower concern for money may translate directly into practice. Women's lower charges may also reflect the fact that women are more likely than men to take salaried jobs that pay physicians less for medical procedures, another indication of women's lower interest in money. Despite an expected liberal contribution to the profession of medicine, women may be slightly less likely to work in free clinics. Women's progressive ideals may not be as important as personal considerations when deciding how much volunteer work they will do.

Although women may have some impact on their colleagues, medical education, and health care, it is not proposed that they will radically change the power structure of the medical profession. The optimism thus far presented about the possible consequences of the recent increase of women in medicine must be counterbalanced with the following cautions: women continue to be such a small minority of the total physicians in this country (about 10 percent)[6] that their impact will be limited; women physicians in the past have been in lower status positions in the profession and thus have not had access to power, influence, or decision-making networks; and class and professional loyalties may prove stronger than women's sympathies with lower status groups.

Prejudice against Women
Physicians and Patients

As expected, Table 7.3 shows that women were much more sensitive than men to specific issues concerning discrimination against women physicians and patients during both freshman and senior year. Among freshmen, women acknowledged the pressure on women physicians to choose traditionally female fields and to avoid traditionally male fields (58.3 percent), the need for more women doctors (95.8 percent), and the patronizing and prejudicial way that physicians treat

TABLE 7.3

Means, Standard Deviations, and Percentage Distributions on Measures concerning the Treatment of Women Physicians and Patients for Males and Females during Their Freshman and Senior Years in Medical School, 1975 and 1978 (with correlation coefficients between measures across time and T-tests for dependent samples)

Variable	Freshman Year, 1975					Senior Year, 1978						
	Index Score[a]		Percentage in Each Category			Index Score		Percentage in Each Category				
	Mean	Standard Deviation	Disagree	Neutral	Agree	Mean	Standard Deviation	Disagree	Neutral	Agree	T-Test	r
There is professional and public prejudice against women physicians												
Male	2.95	.91	38.6	24.6	36.7	2.87	1.04	43.0	21.7	35.3	.97	.31
Female	3.14	.91	26.4	27.8	45.8	3.05	1.03	36.1	22.2	41.7	.55	.08
There is pressure on women physicians to choose certain fields, such as pediatrics												
Male	3.08[b]	.83	25.6	37.2	37.2	2.95[b]	1.11	38.6	20.8	40.6	1.51	.24
Female	3.54	.98	16.7	25.0	58.3	3.75	1.08	18.1	18.1	63.9	1.38	.25
There is a need for more women physicians in this country												
Male	3.77[b]	.92	14.0	12.6	73.4	3.53[b]	1.00	19.3	19.8	60.9	4.00[c]	.60
Female	4.64	.54	1.4	2.8	95.8	4.53	.67	4.2	1.4	94.4	1.24	.32
Physicians generally treat women patients in a patronizing and prejudicial way												
Male	2.89[b]	.62	33.3	47.8	18.8	2.85[b]	.83	43.5	30.4	26.1	.65	.40
Female	3.46	.79	13.9	27.8	58.3	3.86	.86	8.3	19.4	72.2	3.62[c]	.36

r = correlation coefficient

[a] All variables are indexes composed of two or more questionnaire items calculated on 207 males and 72 females. The range of possible values is one to five for all measures. Scores of 1.0 to 2.50 are labeled "disagree," scores of 2.51 to 3.49 are labeled "neutral," and scores of 3.50 to 5.0 are labeled "agree."

[b] Indicates a $p < .01$ of a significant difference between the male and female means using a one-tailed T-test.

[c] Indicates a $p < .01$ of a significant difference in orientation from freshman to senior year on a two-tailed T-test.

female patients (58.3 percent) to a much greater extent than the males (37.2 percent, 73.4 percent and 18.8 percent, respectively). Although women tended to agree more than men that medicine was harder for women because of professional and public prejudice against women physicians, the sex difference on this variable was not significant. It seems that women were aware of prejudice against their sex, but they were somewhat more hesitant to acknowledge any handicaps associated with discrimination.*

Part of the substantial sex differences on women's issues during freshman year were due to the low saliency of many issues for men. Table 7.4 shows that men were much more likely to hold no opinion (ranging from 30 percent to 56 percent) than women (ranging from 11 percent to about 28 percent) on items in the indexes concerning specialty choice pressure on women physicians and the prejudicial treatment of female patients. Both males and females were most likely to express a neutral opinion about whether gynecologists have an accurate view of female sexuality. This is an issue that many students, especially men, had no experience with before medical school. Having been patients, it is not surprising that females were more aware of the patronizing treatment that women patients experience. Before entering medical school, it also seems likely that women would have anticipated some of the prejudicial conditions (such as specialty choice pressure) due to the sometimes biased expectations of family and friends, talking with women in medicine, and reading about sexism in the medical profession. Thus it appeared that, upon entrance to medical school, male medical students were unaware of specific instances of sex discrimination in the profession, whereas females were in substantial agreement that prejudicial treatment exists.

During senior year the percentage of students holding no opinion on the women's issues shown in Table 7.4 decreased dramatically (men ranging from about 10 to 30 percent and women ranging from

---

*The lack of a statistically significant sex difference in freshman year on the index concerning professional and public prejudice against women physicians reflects a sampling problem. The sex difference on this variable was originally significant on the 326 students who answered the first questionnaire. Owing to slight variations in the male and female means for the subset of the sample answering both questionnaires, the sex difference is no longer significant. Initially, however, the sex difference on the index concerning professional and public prejudice against women physicians was smaller than the sex difference on any other women's issue.

TABLE 7.4

Percentage Distributions on Items concerning Specialty Choice Pressure on Women Physicians and the Prejudicial Treatment of Female Patients for Males and Females during Their Freshman and Senior Years in Medical School, 1975 and 1978

	Percentage in Each Category								Neutral to Disagree	Neutral to Agree*	Number
	Freshman Year, 1975				Senior Year, 1978						
Indexes and Items	Disagree	Neutral	Agree	Number	Disagree	Neutral	Agree	Number			
There is pressure on women physicians to choose certain fields, such as pediatrics											
Pressure on women to specialize in some fields like pediatrics											
Male	21.5	42.4	36.1	205	15.5	52.2	32.4	207	51	29	89
Female	23.6	19.4	56.9	72	2.8	33.8	63.4	71	50	50	14
Women discouraged from specializing in some fields like surgery											
Male	24.9	42.9	32.2	205	9.8	33.7	56.6	205	27	64	90
Female	18.3	19.7	62.0	71	1.4	15.3	83.3	72	27	67	15
Physicians generally treat women patients in a patronizing and prejudicial way											
Gynecologists treat female patients without respect											
Male	57.8	30.1	12.1	206	11.2	58.0	30.7	205	53	29	62
Female	43.1	12.5	44.4	72	2.8	31.0	66.2	71	33	56	9
Male doctors are patronizing to female patients											
Male	26.7	37.4	35.9	206	12.6	49.0	38.3	206	47	36	78
Female	18.1	22.2	59.7	72	8.3	22.2	69.4	72	31	44	16
Male doctors are not sensitive to female patients											
Male	32.2	32.2	35.6	205	10.7	46.8	42.4	205	37	46	68
Female	16.7	11.1	72.2	72	4.2	12.5	83.3	72	12	62	8
Gynecology has an inaccurate view of female sexuality											
Male	21.0	56.1	22.9	205	30.4	37.3	32.4	204	37	27	117
Female	11.1	27.8	61.1	72	13.9	9.7	76.4	72	10	75	20

*"Neutral to Disagree" refers to freshmen who started school with no opinion on an item and ended up disagreeing in the senior year. "Neutral to Agree" refers to freshmen who started school with no opinion on an item and ended up agreeing in the senior year.

Note: All items are percentaged across the rows so that categories "Disagree," "Neutral," and "Agree" sum to approximately 100 percent. Deviations from 100 percent are due to rounding. The category "Disagree" includes somewhat and strongly disagree. The category "Agree" includes somewhat and strongly agree. Neutral indicates a no-opinion response. Number refers to the number of valid cases.

154

about 1 to 14 percent). The presence of women in medical school probably contributed to the increased saliency of these discrimination issues for both sexes. As shown in Table 7.4, however, holding an opinion did not always mean becoming more aware of discrimination.

Table 7.3 indicates that sex differences on issues concerning the treatment of women physicians and patients persisted to senior year. In contrast to the men, women continued to be more conscious of specialty choice pressure on women physicians, the need for more women doctors, and the patronizing treatment of female patients. Furthermore, Table 7.4 shows that, among seniors, both males and females were more likely to agree that women were discouraged from specializing in surgery (56.6 percent and 83.3 percent of the men and women, respectively) than to acknowledge the pressure on women to choose pediatrics (32.4 percent and 63.4 percent of the men and women, respectively). During freshman year, neither males nor females made a distinction between pressure to choose pediatrics and not to select surgery; yet, by senior year both sexes had become more aware of the taboo placed on women who choose surgery. In fact, in a recent study of medical school graduates from 1960 to 1978, the small percentage of women selecting surgery remained stable, whereas the large proportion in pediatrics had declined somewhat. [7] The values of seniors in North Carolina were therefore reflecting what may be a change in specialty choice pressure, that is, less pressure on women to choose pediatrics despite a continued stigma on choosing surgery.*

The low correlations over time shown in Table 7.3 for men and especially women on women's indexes and the few significant differences in the means across time indicate less overall group change than individual fluctuation. It seems useful to determine the pattern of change over time for males and females because the means mask much individual fluctuation. Table 7.5 shows the percentages of males and females that began medical school with a high score on indexes concerning women physicians and patients (those in the category

---

*The percentage of seniors agreeing to the two items contained in the index concerning specialty choice pressure on women (see Table 7.4) appears somewhat inflated when compared with the percentage agreeing on the index (see Table 7.3). Because the index scores are the average of the responses on both items, those who responded by agreeing to one item and disagreeing to the other end up in the middle category on the index. Indexes can be somewhat misleading because those who score in the middle category include those with no opinion on the items as well as those with conflicting views on the items.

TABLE 7.5

Percentage Distributions Showing Changes in Attitude on Measures concerning the Treatment of Women Physicians and Patients among Males and Females in Medical School, 1975 to 1978

| | Measures concerning the Treatment of Women | | | | | | | |
| | Bias toward Women Doctors | | Specialty Choice Pressure | | Need More Women Doctors | | Bias toward Women Patients | |
Attitudinal Change	Percent	Number	Percent	Number	Percent	Number	Percent	Number
Started with a high score ("agree") and ended with a lower score[a]								
Male	51	76	51	77	25	152	49	39
Female	52	33	33	42	4	69	26	42
Started with a low score ("disagree") and ended with a higher score[b]								
Male	38	80	40	53	41	29	38	69
Female	63	19	83	12	100	1	70	10

[a]This category includes those who started medical school agreeing with these women's issues (those in the category "agree" in Table 7.3) and as seniors did not agree (ended in categories "neutral" or "disagree").

[b]This category includes those who started medical school disagreeing with these women's issues (those in category "disagree" in Table 7.3) and as seniors ended up more positive (in categories "neutral" or "agree").

Note: All percentages are based on the number given. The omitted percentages refer to all those who did not undergo attitudinal change.

"agree" in Table 7.3) and as seniors had a lower score (categories "neutral" or "disagree"). Likewise, this table also shows those who started with a low score on women's issues ("disagree") but ended with a higher score ("neutral" or "agree"). Because of the small number of cases in some of the cells of the table, we must be cautious about relying too much on these data. The table does, however, suggest a different pattern of change for males and females.

Among the students who came to medical school expecting a great deal of discrimination, many apparently found conditions better than they expected; their scores on women's indexes went down over time. This was especially true for men so that as a group they were more likely than women to leave school with the feeling that sexism had decreased or at least was not as problematic as expected. Because of recent improvements for women in medicine and of less overt discrimination, the decreased concern over sexism may reflect some actual changes. Among the women who as freshmen felt that sexism was an issue in medicine, most continued to feel this way despite any improvements. Although very few women came to medical school denying the existence of sex discrimination in medicine, those who did were more likely to raise their consciousness about women's issues than were men who came with similar attitudes.

Looking back at Table 7.4, we see that on women's issues where many students began with a neutral opinion, the experience in medical school led to some students becoming more sympathetic and some becoming less sympathetic with the problems of women. Although the number of females who started with a neutral opinion was small, these women tended to become more aware of discrimination than their male peers who also began with no opinion on these women's issues. Thus, the trends over time point to some polarization between the sexes on these women's issues, with women as a group becoming more aware of some of these issues and men tending to become slightly less sensitive. Examining the differences between the male and female means in Table 7.3 tends to support this conclusion because these differences tend to be somewhat larger during the senior year than during the freshman year. Although the experience in medical school seems to raise the consciousness concerning sexism in medicine of some students, it tends to do this more for females than for males.

The author had expected that the presence of women in medical school would raise the consciousness of their male peers. Although for some this has apparently happened, a reversal or backlash in opinion also appears to have been a trend. A backlash effect was also noted by researchers studying women managers in two companies so that the business with the larger proportion of women had more of a problem with sex discrimination.[8] This backlash trend is echoed in the following statements made during interviews with two female medical students.

Women are acting differently and some of the men are
just real threatened by it and I think this backlash is
part of the conservatism. The white male is probably
real pissed off. He's not quite as dominant as he used
to be. [University of North Carolina]

Most of the women in our class are not real gung ho out-
going feminists. There are a few that are really out-
going feminists . . . but that has played an important
part in turning off the males in our class. The majority of males are very much opposed to the feminist movement and I've seen that evolve 'cause most of them
didn't have any opinion of it when they came here.
Through this contact with these few girls they have gotten
to have a negative attitude. [Bowman Gray]

The sentiments expressed by two male medical students are consistent with the interpretation given by the two females.

A lot of the girls were very, very vocal and outspoken on
various issues, E. R. A. , smoking, things of this nature
and I think that they stirred up a lot of ill feelings. So
people may not look at female medical students as favorably now. [Bowman Gray]

Among the male members of our class there is a certain amount of sarcastic dislike for some of the more
outspoken women in our class. There was always a kind
of teasing or chauvinism issue. At the same time there
has been a sort of slow and steady growing undercurrent
of realizing that women have just as vital role in medicine as men do. That's been good. I think the bellig-
erence that sometimes comes on with women that feel
very strongly about the issues . . . has had a very negative effect on men and just on the whole atmosphere
here. It creates tension and it has created a wall of sep-
aration. . . . Women have been very chauvinistic about
their stance and been very unbudging, and that has created
a wall of tension and anger. [Duke]

Because women have shown more concern than men with discrimination toward women, it seems likely that their presence has
contributed to and will in the future contribute to improved conditions
for women in medicine. Although vocal women may have a negative
effect on some of their colleagues, they also appear to have heightened
others' awareness and may have been an impetus for eliminating sex-

ism in medicine. Conditions for women patients also may improve if in addition to being more egalitarian in treating patients, women physicians serve as nonsexist role models for other physicians. In fact, at the University of North Carolina in 1976, a few first-year women medical students helped to initiate and organize a program with a local women's health cooperative to train medical students to do gynecological examinations with greater sensitivity to the needs of female patients. This program has now expanded so that women in the Women's Health Teaching Group (as the group is now called) who have been trained in self-examination, self-help, and women's health issues are being paid to teach the technical as well as psychological and social aspects of the pelvic examination to medical students, physician assistants, nurse practitioners, and even physicians. The Women's Health Teaching Group is composed of women medical students and women from the local community who are in a variety of occupations (not all health related), all of whom are interested in the quality of women's health care. A preliminary study on medical students at the University of North Carolina and favorable reports from the faculty at that school have suggested that this ongoing pelvic teaching program has made them more aware of female patients' needs and has provided an egalitarian alternative to the traditional gynecological examination. [9] Another study indicates that women medical students at Harvard have also been responsible for initiating a pelvic teaching program at their school similar to the one in North Carolina. [10] If women medical students at all schools initiate such innovative improvements in medical education, they may help eliminate the patronizing and prejudicial treatment of women patients in the future. The fact that women medical students have helped organize and continue to be involved with such an innovative teaching program lends some support to the contention that values may have relevant implications for behavior.

Furthermore, women medical students, physicians, and other women health professionals have begun to initiate conferences throughout the country (sponsored by the American Medical Women's Association and the American Medical Association) to discuss the problems of women in medicine. One such conference was organized by three women medical students at Duke Medical School in the fall of 1980 in order to discuss strategies for increasing women's leadership in medicine and for improving the profession's treatment of minority women. Some of the goals deemed worthwhile for the coming years were working on the passage of the Equal Rights Amendment in North Carolina; helping medical students and housestaff develop ways to reduce stress; working to increase minority admissions into medical school; getting the faculty to allow the Women's Health Teaching Group to do pelvic examination instruction at Duke; improving patient care; and establishing communication networks among women physicians, women allied health professionals, and minority women in medicine. These conferences organized by medical students to stimulate reforms in medicine are further evidence that women will have a liberalizing effect on the profession of medicine and medical education.

Physician Maldistribution

Initially, the author predicted a few sex differences on plans to practice in need areas and specialties. Men were expected to choose rural practice more than women, whereas women were expected to prefer inner-city practice more than men. Among first-year students, men were slightly more oriented to rural practice, as shown in Table 7.6, but this sex difference was not significant. In the freshman year, men expressed a greater commitment than women to choosing a specialty and geographic area that need physicians, but they were not more likely to actually plan a practice in a need area or specialty. In fact, as expected, first-year women were somewhat more inclined to plan an inner-city ghetto practice (32.0 percent) than first-year men (21.3 percent).

Although over time students as a whole became much less committed to patient-need practices, females remained more interested in inner-city ghetto practice (22.2 percent) compared with the males (12.6 percent). Because both males' and females' interests in ghetto practice decreased comparably in four years, the original sex difference on this practice plan persisted through senior year. When asked, however, the type of location in which they will most likely work, only one male and one female in the whole sample chose inner-city ghetto practice. Although women maintained more interest in ghetto practice over time, neither sex saw this need area as their most likely option. Women's greater interest in ghetto practice probably reflects their more liberal values and is consistent with national data on 1978 U.S. medical school graduates. [11]

All students were less interested in rural practice in their senior year; however, males decreased slightly less than females on this practice plan. Therefore, males expressed slightly more interest in rural practice as seniors (36.0 percent) than was shown by females (29.2 percent). Perhaps locating in a rural area was seen by women as more socially and personally limiting, a topic discussed more fully in the next chapter.

In the senior year, the sexes did not differ in their plans to practice primary-care medicine or in their stated commitment to choosing a specialty and geographic area that need physicians. Ac-

TABLE 7.6

Means, Standard Deviations, and Percentage Distributions on Measures concerning Physician Maldistribution for Males and Females during Their Freshman and Senior Years in Medical School, 1975 and 1978
(with correlation coefficients between measures across time and T-tests for dependent samples)

| | Freshman Year, 1975 | | | | | Senior Year, 1978 | | | | | | |
| | Index Score[a] | | Percentage in Each Category | | | Index Score | | Percentage in Each Category | | | | |
Variable	Mean	Standard Deviation	Disagree	Neutral	Agree	Mean	Standard Deviation	Disagree	Neutral	Agree	T-Test	r
Expect to practice primary-care medicine												
Male	3.83	1.12	18.8	8.2	72.9	3.22	1.56	42.5	7.7	49.8	5.86	.41
Female	3.92	1.15	18.1	9.7	72.2	3.32	1.42	34.7	11.1	54.2	3.57	.39
Expect a rural practice												
Male	2.58	1.00	43.0	—	57.0	2.13[c]	1.04	64.0	—	36.0	6.33	.50
Female	2.49	1.01	52.8	—	47.2	1.88	0.93	70.8	—	29.2	5.04	.44
Expect an inner-city ghetto practice												
Male	1.89[d]	0.78	78.7	—	21.3	1.46[d]	0.74	87.4	—	12.6	7.99	.50
Female	2.18	0.78	68.1	—	32.0	1.72	0.94	77.8	—	22.2	3.98	.36
Committed to choosing a specialty and geographic area that need physicians												
Male	3.68[c]	1.00	18.8	16.9	64.3	3.15	1.26	39.1	17.9	43.0	7.05	.56
Female	3.39	1.16	27.8	20.8	51.4	3.01	1.24	38.9	25.0	36.1	2.78	.53

r = correlation coefficient

[a]Variables are indexes composed of two or more questionnaire items with the exception of rural practice and inner-city ghetto practice expectations, which are single-item measures. Calculations are based on 207 cases for males and 72 cases for females, with the exception of the single-item measures computed on slightly fewer cases. The range of possible values is one to five for all measures except for the single-item variables that range from one to four. On indexes ranging from one to five, scores of 1.0 to 2.50 are labeled "disagree," scores of 2.51 to 3.49 are labeled "neutral," and scores of 3.50 to 5.0 are labeled "agree." On single-item measures coded from one to four, responses of "very unlikely" and "somewhat unlikely" are labeled "disagree," and "very likely" and "somewhat likely" are labeled "agree."

[b]All T-tests have a p < .01 of a significant difference in orientation from freshman to senior year using a two-tailed T-test.

[c]Indicates a p < .05 of a significant difference between the male and female means using a one-tailed T-test.

[d]Indicates a p < .01 of a significant difference between the male and female means using a one-tailed T-test.

cording to national data on all senior medical students in 1978, 59.1 percent of the women planned primary-care careers compared with 55.9 percent of the men. [12] Data collected here on students in North Carolina seem fairly comparable to national data. Furthermore, men and women were fairly equally distributed in the primary-care fields in the senior year so that women did not choose a specialty in pediatrics substantially more than the men (11.3 percent of the women compared to 7.8 percent of the men).* As noted before, pressure on females to choose pediatrics seems to be waning. We might have expected women to plan a primary-care practice much more than the men because this is typically the field for those oriented to helping people and to close patient relationships. There was a correlation of .40 in the senior year between planning a primary-care practice and viewing helping people as an important part of one's medical career. Since primary-care medicine tends to involve long hours and inflexible schedules, women may choose a less demanding field as a result of anticipating time pressures involved with raising a family or because of pressures from a spouse for those already married.

Thus, professional socialization appeared to have a similar effect on the location and specialty choices of men and women; both became less interested in patient-need practices. Professional socialization was not strong enough to wipe out the original sex differences on planning an inner-city ghetto practice. Personal considerations probably dictated women's decreasing interest in rural practices as much as professional socialization.

The increase in the proportion of women in medicine should not have too great an overall impact on the problem of physician maldistribution. Although women may be slightly more responsive to the need for physicians in the inner-city, they also appear to be somewhat less likely to serve in rural areas. As we have seen in Chapter 6, other background variables (such as rural origins) appear to be more important than gender in predicting commitment to geographic and specialty areas of patient need.

SUMMARY

Compared with males, females began medical school somewhat more oriented to humanitarian patient-care values, political and economic change in the profession of medicine, the problems facing women physicians and patients, and inner-city ghetto practice. Through training, women remained more interested in most of these issues and

---

*These percentages are based on 71 females and 205 males who responded to the open-ended item, "Which field do you think you actually will be working in ten years from now?"

career plans and became more concerned with egalitarian patient care. During senior year, however, men were more likely than women to consider rural practice and to plan volunteer work, probably reflecting personal considerations more than differences in professional socialization between the sexes.

Both males and females have come closer through training to adopting traditional professional views, that is, political and economic status quo in the organization of medicine and geographic and specialty choice based on personal and professional interests rather than patient need. Socialization appeared to have a similar influence on both men and women; medical student status (or anticipated physician status) appeared more important than gender in determining much attitudinal change. Despite this increased conservatism among students over time, females continued to advocate more liberal stances on political and economic issues and remained slightly more committed to an inner-city ghetto practice because they started school that way. Thus, professional socialization was not a great leveler of attitudinal variation because it has not been strong enough to wipe out or reduce most initial sex differences on these orientations. Professional orientation differences between the sexes in the senior year seem to result from the selection process into medical school more than from the socialization process in school.

Originally, the author proposed that medical school might have a less conservative influence on women than on men. This appears to be the case only on some issues related to sex discrimination and to the egalitarian treatment of patients. Women have been more likely than men to remain sensitive to sexism in medicine and to become critical of physicians' judgments and concerned with giving patients health information. These findings lend limited support to the hypothesis that professional socialization in medical school has a differential effect on the sexes.

Furthermore, interviews conducted with a limited number of medical students suggest that women's militancy in medical school on issues of sex discrimination has resulted in some men becoming more aware of sexism and some becoming part of a conservative backlash. The data presented in this chapter has shown some polarization between the sexes on issues of sex discrimination, apparently an unfortunate side effect of the women's movement.

Although the potential implications of the findings for the profession, medical education, and health care are limited to the extent that students' professional orientations may not predict subsequent behavior, these findings are suggestive. The controversial issue of whether attitudes are useful in predicting future behavior is discussed in the last chapter. Because women have been more committed than men to humanitarian and nonauthoritarian values with patients, they may develop more egalitarian relationships with their patients in practice, marked by better communication and rapport. Because some of the worst complaints leveled at the medical profession have concerned the doctor/patient relationship, the increase in the proportion of women in medicine may add a needed touch of humanity to the practice of medicine.

Because women have shown more concern than men about discrimination toward women, it seems likely that their presence has contributed to and will in the future contribute to improved conditions for women medical students and physicians. Conditions for women patients may also improve if, in addition to being more egalitarian in treating patients, women physicians serve as nonsexist role models for other physicians.

Women's greater likelihood of advocating reforms like socialized medicine and lower physician income may translate in practice to charging lower fees than men and to being more responsive to public health needs. Women's lower interest in money does not mean, however, that they will do more volunteer work in free clinics. To the contrary, men plan slightly more hours of volunteer work than women. Women's orientation to political and economic change suggests that they will have a liberalizing effect on the profession of medicine. Although women may have some impact on their colleagues, medical education, and health care, it is not proposed that they will radically change the power structure of the medical profession.

This book began with a quote from one participant at a recent conference on women in medicine who cautioned that there has been a "prior assumption that if we increase the number of women in medicine this will have a . . . beneficial effect on the health care of men and women, and . . . improve the quality of the health care provided by women physicians and by men physicians. But we do not actually know that this is going to happen."[13] Evidence has been given in this chapter that suggests that women may have a positive impact on health care and the profession of medicine as long as the women selected into medical school continue to be more liberal and humanitarian than the men.

NOTES

1. See, for example, Janet M. Cuca, "The Specialization and Career Preferences of Women and Men Recently Graduated from U.S. Medical Schools," Journal of the American Medical Women's Association 34 (November 1979): 425-35; Daniel H. Funkenstein, Medical Students, Medical Schools and Society During Five Eras: Factors Affecting the Career Choices of Physicians 1958-1976 (Cambridge, Mass.: Ballinger, 1978), pp. 73-82; and Marilyn Heins, "Career and Life Patterns of Women and Men Physicians," in Becoming a Physi-

cian, ed. Eileen C. Shapiro and Leah M. Lowenstein (Cambridge, Mass.: Ballinger, 1979), pp. 217-35.

2. George E. Dickinson and Algene A. Pearson, "Sex Differences of Physicians in Relating to Dying Patients," Journal of the American Medical Women's Association 34 (January 1979): 45-47.

3. Mary Fruen, Arthur Rothman, and Jan Steiner, "Comparison of Characteristics of Male and Female Medical School Applicants," Journal of Medical Education 49 (February 1974): 137-45; Funkenstein, Medical Students, Medical Schools and Society, pp. 73-82; John Kosa and Robert E. Coker, Jr., "The Female Physician in Public Health: Conflict and Reconciliation of the Sex and Professional Roles," in Professional Woman, ed. Athena Theodore (Cambridge, Mass.: Schenkman, 1971), pp. 195-206; and Robert Roessler, Forrest Collins, and Roy B. Mefferd, "Sex Similarities in Successful Medical School Applicants," Journal of the American Medical Women's Association 30 (June 1975): 254-65.

4. Cuca, "Specialization and Career Preferences," pp. 425-35; Funkenstein, Medical Students, Medical Schools and Society, pp. 73-82; Kosa and Coker, "Female Physician in Public Health," pp. 195-206; and Nancy G. Kutner and Donna R. Brogan, "The Decision to Enter Medicine: Motivations, Social Support, and Discouragements for Women," Psychology of Women Quarterly 5 (Winter 1980): 341-58.

5. Jean W. Adams, "Patient Discrimination against Women Physicians," Journal of the American Medical Women's Association 32 (July 1977): 255-61.

6. Lorna E. Wunderman, Physician Distribution and Medical Licensure in the U.S., 1978 (Monroe, Wis.: American Medical Association, 1979), pp. 13-40.

7. Cuca, "Specialization and Career Preferences," pp. 425-35.

8. Anne Harlan and Carol Weiss, "Sex Differences in Factors Affecting Managerial Career Advancement," Working Paper of the Center for Research on Women, Wellsley College, Wellsley, Mass., 1980.

9. Jane Leserman and Cynthia S. Luke, "An Evaluation of an Innovative Approach to Teaching the Pelvic Examination to Medical Students," presented at the Southern Sociological Society annual meetings, Louisville, Kentucky, April 1981.

10. J. Andrew Billings and John D. Stoeckle, "Pelvic Examination Instruction and the Doctor-Patient Relationship," Journal of Medical Education 52 (October 1977): 834-39.

11. Janet M. Cuca, "1978 U.S. Medical School Graduates: Practice Setting Preferences, Other Career Plans, and Personal Characteristics," Journal of Medical Education 55 (May 1980): 465-68.

12. Cuca, "Specialization and Career Preferences," pp. 425-35.

13. John Walsh, "Summary of the Conference," in Women in Medicine—1976, ed. Carolyn Spieler (New York: Josiah Macy, Jr. Foundation, 1977), p. 78.

8

EXPLAINING SEX DIFFERENCES

In the previous chapter, men's and women's professional orientations were compared in their first and last year of medical school. Data showed that women began and finished their training somewhat more oriented to most values and expectations concerning humanitarian patient care, political and economic change in medicine, the problems facing women physicians and patients, and inner-city ghetto practice. Furthermore, women left school with more egalitarian patient-care values, although men finished with greater interest in rural practice and volunteer work. This chapter will explore why women and men differed initially upon entrance to medical school and why they changed differently on some orientations over time.

Most sociological studies comparing males and females make little attempt to go beyond a simple description of sex differences. We are left wondering what it is about growing up and being a male or female that leads to these sex variations. In this study, attributes associated with early socialization including traditional sex-role socialization will be tested as possible explanations for why women begin medical school with more liberal and humanitarian values and career plans than men. Therefore, the sex differences in professional orientations are expected to be at least partially explained by differences between men and women in personality, political outlook, and the importance they attach to money and status. Women's anticipated minority status in the profession and the liberalizing effect of the women's liberation movement are proposed as residual explanations of initial sex differences in orientation.

In the previous chapter, data pointed to the emergence during medical training of some new sex differences in professional orientations (for example, on egalitarian patient-care values) and the widening of some initial ones (for example, on women's issues). In this chapter, explanations accounting for the differential socialization of men and women will also be tested. A less orderly socialization of women in medical school was expected owing to the isolation and discrimination experienced by women in a male profession, the scarcity of female and patient-oriented role models, and the formation of alternative women's reference groups and minority organizations that reinforce liberal values. This chapter begins by addressing the question of why the sexes begin medical school with different professional values and expectations.

WHY SEX DIFFERENCES IN FIRST-YEAR ORIENTATIONS?

The following variables were examined in this study for their possible role in accounting for initial sex differences in professional orientations: (1) personality characteristics including nurturance (being helpful and sympathetic), dominance (being influential and assertive), competitiveness, and cynicism (believing most people try to use others); (2) general political outlook (liberalism); and (3) choosing medicine for the status and financial rewards. Path analysis and multiple regression techniques were utilized to determine the extent to which the initial sex differences in professional orientation were explained by these selected characteristics associated with primary socialization. The path model specifies the causal ordering of the variables and thus implies a theory explaining sex differences in professional orientations. The utility of the model depends on the validity of the theory that specifies the causal sequence among the variables.

Figure 8.1 shows the basic path model used to obtain estimates of the effects of sex and explanatory variables on professional values and expectations.* Only professional values and expectations that have shown significant sex differences are examined using the path model. A causal ordering of variables is indicated in Figure 8.1. Without longitudinal data on attitude formation before medical school, the theory specifying the causal sequence among variables cannot be

---

*It shows a recursive path model, that is, the causal flow is unidirectional. The four letters U, V, W, and X in the path model indicate residual, unmeasured variables, that is, variables not in the model that might account for variation in the professional orientation measures. They are assumed to be uncorrelated with each other, except for U and V, which reflect unanalyzed correlations between same-stage variables.

FIGURE 8.1

Causal Model for Explaining Sex Differences on Professional Orientation Measures upon Entrance to Medical School

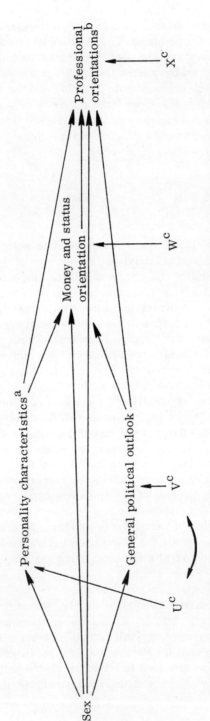

[a]Personality characteristics include nurturance, dominance, competitiveness, and cynicism.

[b]Professional orientations include the following: social and psychological factors are important in health care, choosing medicine in order to help people, profession's control over health should be reduced, favoring a National Service Corps, the health-care system needs to be changed, physicians' status and financial rewards need to be lowered, expect to work for political and social change, pressure on women to choose certain fields, need for more women physicians, women patients treated in patronizing way, plan inner-city practice, and commitment to a specialty and geographic area of need.

[c]U, V, W, and X indicate residual variables, that is, variables not in the model that might account for variation in the professional orientation measures.

tested. Interviews with medical students and logical considerations, however, provide reasonable support for the causal order of variables in the model. Although all variables are measured at one point in time, the development of general personality characteristics and political outlook is assumed to occur prior to the formulation of more specific values and expectations concerning the medical profession. It seems reasonable to assume that general orientations reflecting early socialization are acquired before more specific orientations concerning medicine. Because no causal direction is indicated between same-stage explanatory variables (for example, political outlook, nurturance, and dominance), these correlations are not analyzed in the path model. Furthermore, because choosing medicine for the money and status can be linked to the development of pecuniary values during sex-role socialization, this orientation probably develops prior to other more specific values and expectations concerning medicine. Because this money and status orientation measure refers specifically to one's choice of medicine as a career, it is specified after political outlook and personality attributes that are more generalized. (Choosing medicine for the money and status has been included as an explanatory variable since some argue that women support and are less threatened by economic reforms in medicine—such as socialized medicine or less money for doctors—because they are less interested in money and have less pressure to make it. To test this hypothesis, choosing medicine for the money and status has been included as an explanatory variable in the path model.) Finally, because sex is fixed at birth, it is placed first in the model.

The path model does not include other background variables that might explain variations on professional orientations, because their inclusion would not help elucidate the relationship between sex and these orientations. In other words, this analysis is not aimed at finding all the reasons why people differ in their orientations upon entrance to school but only why males and females appear to differ. As mentioned previously, the sex effects persist and are virtually unchanged by other background variables. Including the background variables in the model would, therefore, not contribute to our understanding of why the sexes differed initially.

It was expected that sex would correlate with the personality traits and with the orientation to money and status because these values are to some extent reflections of traditional sex-role socialization. In addition, women were expected to be more liberal than men because medicine is a deviant career choice for women and a mainstream career path for men. Table 8.1 shows the significant correlations of explanatory variables with sex and with the professional orientations on which the sexes initially differed. As expected, women scored somewhat higher on nurturance and liberalism and were slightly

TABLE 8.1

Statistically Significant Correlations of Sex and Professional Orientation Measures with Explanatory Variables during Medical Students' Freshman Year, 1975

| | Explanatory Variables | | | | | |
| | Personality Characteristics | | | | | Money and |
Professional Orientation Measures and Sex	Nurturance	Dominance	Competitiveness	Cynicism	Liberalism	Status Are Important
Social/psychological important	.28			-.21		.11
Helping people important	.46			-.15		
Reduce profession's control		-.10			.45	-.18
Favor National Service Corps			-.13		.27	-.19
No profits in health care			-.10		.24	-.12
Lower doctor's income	.13	-.17	-.17	-.25	.30	-.39
Money and status are important	-.12	.11		.24	-.13	1.00
Work for political change	.13				.39	
Specialty choice pressure exists			-.15		.21	
Need more women doctors	.17		-.11	-.18	.35	-.11
Bias toward women patients exists	.10		-.15	-.11	.27	-.21
Plan inner-city practice	.20			-.11	.20	
Committed to patient need	.25			-.17		-.14
Sex*	.24			-.11	.17	-.14

*Sex is coded so that zero equals male and one equals female.

Note: The table reports statistically significant correlations at the .05 level or lower. The number of valid cases ranges from 265 to 279 as a result of missing data.

less cynical and oriented to money and status. Contrary to expectation, no significant sex difference was found on dominance and competitiveness; the former was a quality that most students possessed (68.5 percent).* Getting into medical school is highly competitive and requires some assertiveness; it is not surprising, then, that women do not differ from men on these traits. The sex differences in personality, liberalism, and orientation to money and status were expected to account for at least some of the sex differences in professional orientations.

Although Table 8.1 shows many significant zero-order correlations between explanatory variables and professional orientations, not all the path coefficients for explanatory variables were significant when controlling on sex and other same or prior stage variables. The full path model was simplified for each professional orientation so that only significant path coefficients (at the .05 probability level or lower) are reported. Therefore, explanatory variables were deleted from equations when they did not significantly add to explaining variation on a particular professional orientation controlling on sex and other same or prior stage explanatory variables. Tables 8.2 to 8.5 show which specific explanatory variable effects persisted net of sex and same or prior stage variables in predicting the professional orientations concerning the four health-care problem areas, respectively.†

---

*This percentage refers to those scoring above 2.50 on the dominance index ranging from one to four.

†The regression coefficients in reduced form equations predicting intervening variables are not shown in Tables 8.2 to 8.5. These equations were omitted in order to simplify the presentation of the results and because this information was not considered particularly useful in the present analysis. Because none of the explanatory variables or professional orientation measures were perfectly reliable, the mediating effects were somewhat lower than would be expected if measurement were more precise. Using multiple regression techniques, interaction terms between sex and all explanatory variables were tested for significance. In other words, the author determined if the sex effects were the same for those who scored high compared with those who scored low on the explanatory variables. The few significant interactions were ignored in the analysis because for the most part they were theoretically uninformative, most did not add much to the variance explained on the professional orientation measures, and the number of significant interactions was not much greater than would be expected due to chance.

The terminology used in Tables 8.2 to 8.5 and in the discussion accounting for sex differences needs some explanation. The total sex effect is the beta weight of sex when regressing the dependent variable on sex alone, which is also the zero-order correlation coefficient. Intuitively, it is the importance or strength that sex alone has in predicting a particular professional orientation. The direct sex effect (the sex beta coefficient) is a measure of the importance of sex in predicting a professional orientation when controlling on all explanatory variables in the path model, that is, the part of the total sex effect not explained by other variables in the model. The indirect sex effect is the part of the total sex effect mediated by explanatory variables. It is calculated by subtracting the direct sex effect from the total sex effect.[1] Tables 8.2 to 8.5 also show the proportion of the total sex effect for each orientation mediated by explanatory variables, that is, the extent to which initial sex differences in professional orientations can be accounted for by gender differences in personality, political outlook, and money and status orientation. By entering each same stage explanatory variable last into the equation predicting a professional orientation, we can determine which explanatory variable or variables account most for these sex differences. The results of this procedure are reported in the text.

Physicians' Relationships with Patients

At the beginning of this chapter, the author showed that women begin medical school more oriented to the human side of medicine. The proportion of the total indirect sex effect over the total sex effect shown in Table 8.2 illustrates that women's greater nurturance accounts entirely for their greater emphasis on choosing medicine in order to help people and only partially (24 percent) for their greater emphasis on the social and psychological aspects of health care. The low variance on the index concerning the importance of social and psychological aspects in patient care probably accounts in part for the small mediating effects of the explanatory variables. Thus, compared with men, women are more motivated by altruistic reasons for choosing medicine because they learn early on to value helping people. Beyond being socialized to help others, women traditionally have been taught to place greater value than men on close personal relationships. This is supported by studies of physicians and medical students showing that women are more likely than men to value close patient contacts.[2] Although untested in this study, this general interpersonal orientation of women might partially account for their greater emphasis on empathy and other social and psychological aspects of patient care because women's desires to nurture did not fully explain this sex difference.

TABLE 8.2

Standardized and Metric Regression Coefficients in Equations for a Model Explaining Sex Differences in Professional Orientations concerning the Doctor/Patient Relationship during Medical Students' Freshman Year, 1975

Predictor Variables	Dependent Variables			
	Standardized Coefficients		Unstandardized Coefficients	
Social/Psychological Important				
Sex	.231	.175	.288	.218
Nurturance		.233		.391
R^2	.054	.105		
Constant			4.249	3.083

$$\frac{\text{Total indirect}^a}{\text{Total sex}} = \frac{.056}{.231} = .24$$

Predictor Variables	Standardized Coefficients		Unstandardized Coefficients	
Helping People Important				
Sex	.112	-.001	.148	-.001
Nurturance		.464		.826
R^2	.013	.215		
Constant			3.307	.846

$$\frac{\text{Total indirect}}{\text{Total sex}} = \frac{.113}{.112} = 1.01^b$$

[a] The total indirect sex effect divided by the total sex effect yields the proportion of the initial sex differences in professional orientations, which can be accounted for by gender differences on explanatory variables.

[b] Slight suppressor effect.

Note: Explanatory variables (liberal outlook, nurturance, dominance, cynicism, competitiveness, and money and status orientation) are not in the equations if the path coefficient is not significant at the .05 level or lower, net of sex and other same-stage or prior-stage variables.

Political and Economic Change

As shown previously, women began medical school more supportive of political and economic change in medicine. Table 8.3 shows
that some of their more liberal views toward political and economic
change in medicine were partially accounted for by their more liberal
political sentiments upon entrance to medical school. (The regression
coefficients for sex are reduced when liberal outlook is added to the
equations.) Being less oriented to money and status accounted only
slightly for their more favorable views toward reducing the profession's control over medicine through government intervention, implementing a National Service Corps, and lowering doctors' incomes.
(The regression coefficients for sex are reduced only slightly when
the importance of money and status are added to these equations.)
Thus the argument that women will favor political changes in the profession that may hurt physicians financially because they are less
personally oriented to money and status seems to have only limited
validity. In addition, personality differences between men and women
appear to have accounted very little for the initial sex differences on
political and economic change issues. As indicated in Table 8.3,
the slightly greater cynicism expressed by men when compared with
women accounted only minimally for their more negative view toward
lowering physicians' incomes and to their greater interest in money
and status. Thus sex differences on liberalism appear to explain sex
differences on political and economic change issues more than variations on personality or orientation to money and status.

Women's more liberal political outlook is not explained by any
background differences between the sexes (for example, social class
or race) or by their parents' more liberal outlooks. In other words,
the relationship between sex and general political liberalism persists
when controlling on background variables and on parents' general
political outlook. Perhaps women applying to medical school are more
liberal than men because women are to some extent pioneers in a male
profession. Because medicine is a more deviant career for women
than men, choosing medicine may reflect a less traditional outlook
for women. The author speculates that female medical students generally are more liberal than their male peers in part because of self-
selection.

Table 8.3 shows that only some of the sex differences on political and economic change issues are explained by personality, political outlook, and money and status differences between the sexes
(ranging from 17 percent to 83 percent); therefore, other factors
must also contribute to these sex effects. Having anticipated minority
status and having been exposed to the ideology of the women's movement also may help explain women's more liberal orientation on po-

TABLE 8.3

Standardized and Metric Regression Coefficients in Equations for a Model Explaining Sex Differences in Professional Orientations concerning Political and Economic Change in Medicine during Medical Students' Freshman Year, 1975

Dependent Variables

Predictor Variables	Standardized Coefficients			Unstandardized Coefficients		
Reduce Profession's Control						
Sex	.132	.056	.042	.310	.132	.098
Liberal outlook		.444	.431		.576	.559
Money and status important			-.117			-.203
R^2	.018	.209	.222			
Constant				2.882	.973	1.432
$\dfrac{\text{Total indirect*}}{\text{Total sex}} = \dfrac{.090}{.132} = .68$						
Favor National Service Corps						
Sex	.145	.103	.085	.221	.156	.129
Liberal outlook		.249	.233		.210	.196
Money and status important			-.144			-.161
R^2	.021	.081	.101			
Constant				1.892	1.197	1.562
$\dfrac{\text{Total indirect}}{\text{Total sex}} = \dfrac{.060}{.145} = .41$						
No Profits in Health Care						
Sex	.171	.134		.484	.379	
Liberal outlook		.216			.340	
R^2	.029	.075				
Constant				2.850	1.724	
$\dfrac{\text{Total indirect}}{\text{Total sex}} = \dfrac{.037}{.171} = .22$						

(continued)

175

TABLE 8.3 (continued)

Predictor Variables	Standardized Coefficients			Unstandardized Coefficients		
Dependent Variables						
Lower Doctor's Income						
Sex	.214	.144	.115	.399	.270	.214
Liberal outlook		.261	.232		.270	.240
Dominance		-.170	-.140		-.338	-.278
Cynicism		-.209	-.145		-.411	-.285
Money and status important			-.293			-.404
R^2	.046	.190	.268			
Constant				2.977	3.678	4.213
Total indirect = .099 = .46						
Total sex = .214						
Money and Status Are Important						
Sex	-.143	-.118		-.194	-.160	
Cynicism		.226			.322	
R^2	.020	.071				
Constant				1.991	1.465	
Total indirect = -.025 = .17						
Total sex = -.143						
Work for Political Change						
Sex	.115	.020		.193	.034	
Liberal outlook		.386			.360	
Nurturance		.118			.267	
R^2	.013	.169				
Constant				2.118	.129	
Total indirect = .095 = .83						
Total sex = .115						

*The total indirect sex effect divided by the total sex effect yields the proportion of the initial sex differences in professional orientation, which can be accounted for by gender differences on explanatory variables.

Note: Explanatory variables (liberal outlook, nurturance, dominance, cynicism, competitiveness, and money and status orientation) are not in the equations if the path coefficient is not significant at the .05 level or lower, net of sex and other same-stage or prior-stage variables.

litical and economic issues in medicine upon entrance to medical school. As shown in Chapter 6, blacks, another minority group in medicine, also tend to begin medical school with more liberal views on some political changes in the profession. Minority status or anticipated minority status may lead to holding values more conflicting with the status quo.

The author speculates that exposure to the women's movement may have politicized students about issues beyond those relevant only to women. Many of the women's health publications link women's health problems on all levels to the need for restructuring the medical-care system.[3] Perhaps women medical students' greater interest in changing the medical profession is the result of more contact with the women's movement and with its implied criticisms of the health-care system. When women cease to be minorities in medicine and when that career path is no longer an unusual or deviant choice for women, the author expects that the political ideologies of first-year women in medical school will resemble more closely those of their male peers. Furthermore, if the women's movement becomes less salient over time, like other recent social movements, women may no longer be more likely to advocate widespread changes in medicine. In the future, women selected into medical school may identify just as much as men with their anticipated class status as physicians rather than with the interests of minorities and low-income Americans.

Prejudice against Women

Upon entrance to medical school, women also were more aware than men of sexism in medicine. Looking at Table 8.4, we note that for the most part sex differences on issues concerning discrimination against physicians and patients are not explained by personality, political outlook, or money and status orientation. No more than 15 percent of the sex effect on any women's issue is accounted for by explanatory variables. (Note the proportions of total indirect over total sex.) The small part of the initial sex differences on women's issues that can be attributed to explanatory variables is mostly a result of women's greater political liberalism. Differences between the sexes on personality and the importance of money and status generally do not account for much of the initial sex differences on issues of sexism in medicine.

Although not specifically tested, it is reasonable to assume that minority status and the women's liberation movement have sensitized female medical students to the problems experienced by women physicians and patients. As noted in Chapter 7, the sex differences initially on views concerning the pressure on women to choose certain

TABLE 8.4

Standardized and Metric Regression Coefficients in Equations for a Model Explaining Sex Differences in Professional Orientations concerning Prejudice against Women Physicians and Patients during Medical Students' Freshman Year, 1975

Predictor Variables	Dependent Variables			
	Standardized Coefficients		Unstandardized Coefficients	
Specialty Choice Pressure Exists				
Sex	.228	.199	.464	.405
Liberal outlook		.166		.187
Dominance		.130		.283
Competitiveness		-.162		-.123
Cynicism		.122		.261
R^2	.052	.126		
Constant			3.079	1.589

$$\frac{\text{Total indirect*}}{\text{Total sex}} = \frac{.029}{.228} = .13$$

Predictor Variables	Standardized Coefficients		Unstandardized Coefficients	
Need More Women Doctors				
Sex	.415	.354	.866	.740
Liberal outlook		.277		.320
Cynicism		-.118		-.260

R^2	.172	.263		
Constant	3.773	3.134		

$$\frac{\text{Total indirect}}{\text{Total sex}} = \frac{.061}{.415} = .15$$

Bias toward Women Patients Exists

Sex	.353	.316	.299	.573	.514	.485
Liberal outlook		.213	.198		.192	.178
Money and status important			-.142			-.170
R^2	.124	.169	.188			
Constant	2.888	2.251	2.637			

$$\frac{\text{Total indirect}}{\text{Total sex}} = \frac{.054}{.353} = .15$$

R^2 = multiple correlation

*The total indirect sex effect divided by the total sex effect yields the proportion of the initial sex differences in professional orientations, which can be accounted for by gender differences on explanatory variables.

Note: Explanatory variables (liberal outlook, nurturance, dominance, cynicism, competitiveness, and money and status orientation) are not in the equations if the path coefficient is not significant at the .05 level or lower, net of sex and other same-stage or prior-stage variables.

specialties and the patronizing treatment of patients were in part a result of the high no-opinion response of the men. It seems likely that before entering medical school women had more contact with and developed more interest in the women's movement through consciousness raising groups, informal discussions, and literature concerning sexism in all areas of American society. Exposure to the ideology of the women's movement may have increased female students' awareness of specific problems encountered by women professionals and women patients. Men who were familiar and sympathetic with the ideas of the women's movement also may have come to medical school more aware of problems encountered by women in medicine. Furthermore, issues concerning the patronizing treatment of women patients and specialty choice pressure were probably more salient to women partially due to their personal experiences as gynecological patients and as premedical students. Certainly, it was in the self-interests of women to be aware of and to oppose sexism in medicine. It was not in the self-interests of men before starting medical school to advocate affirmative action programs and the increase of women in medicine because that would increase the already stiff competition for entrance into medical school. On the other hand, there was probably some social pressure on men to at least espouse equality between the sexes.

Physician Maldistribution

Although in the first year men expressed a greater commitment than women to practice in an area and field that needed physicians, they were not more likely to actually choose such a practice. In fact, women tended to select inner-city ghetto practice more than the men. Table 8.5 shows that the strength of the relationship between sex and commitment to patient need actually increased when controlling on nurturance and choosing medicine for the money and status. (The coefficients for sex increased when explanatory variables were added to the equations.) In other words, if women in medical school showed the same degree of nurturance and interest in money and status as the men, then men would express an even greater commitment than women to patient need. (This is an example of a suppressor effect, that is, an instance where the relationship between two variables increases when controlling on other variables.) If women entering medical school continue to be more nurturant and less interested in money and status, then the difference between the sexes on patient-need commitment will remain relatively slight.

Upon entrance to medical school, females were more likely to choose inner-city ghetto practice primarily because they were more

TABLE 8.5

Standardized and Metric Regression Coefficients in Equations for a Model Explaining Sex Differences in Professional Orientations concerning Physician Maldistribution during Medical Students' Freshman Year, 1975

Predictor Variables	Dependent Variables	
	Standardized Coefficients	Unstandardized Coefficients
Plan Inner-City Practice		
Sex	.088	.158
Liberal outlook	.185	.184
Nurturance	.177	.429
R²	.163 / .027	.293
Constant		1.889
(Sex total / −.003)	.088	
Committed to Patient Need[b]		
Sex	−.194	−.463
Nurturance	.297	.959
Money and status important	−.136	−.241
R²	.098 / .116	
Constant		3.682
(additional values)	−.121 .285 .015	−.290 .919 −.503 .825 1.421

$$\text{Total indirect}^{a} \Big/ \text{Total sex} = \frac{.075}{.163} = .46$$

[a] The total indirect sex effect divided by the total sex effect yields the proportion of the initial sex differences in professional orientations, which can be accounted for by gender differences on explanatory variables.

[b] Because of suppressor effects, the proportion of indirect to total sex effect is not computed because the total sex effect is negative and the indirect sex effect is positive in value.

Note: Explanatory variables (liberal outlook, nurturance, dominance, cynicism, competitiveness, and money and status orientation) are not in the equations if the path coefficient is not significant at the .05 level, net of sex and other same-stage or prior-stage variables.

liberal and more oriented to helping people than were the men (46 percent of the total sex effect was explained by liberal outlook and nurturance). Committing oneself to a patient-need practice is associated with wanting to help others, whereas considering an inner-city ghetto practice is partially a political decision as well.

EXPLAINING GENDER DIFFERENCES IN PROFESSIONAL SOCIALIZATION

So far this chapter has discussed why the sexes have come to medical school with varying values and expectations. To conclude, the author will briefly explore why the sexes changed uniquely during medical school on some professional orientations. Originally the author predicted that differences in professional orientations between men and women might increase over time because of differences in socialization between the sexes. Participation in minority organizations, exposure to the women's movement, and the isolation of women in medicine because of such things as negative treatment by faculty and negative role models were considered factors that might explain differential socialization. By and large, socialization during medical school seemed to have a fairly uniform effect on both men and women so that students, regardless of sex, tended to become more conservative on political and economic issues and to become less interested in patient-need practices. But the experience in medical school appeared to uniquely affect males and females on issues concerning sexism in medicine and the equalization of the doctor/patient relationship more than on other orientations examined in this study.

The values and expectations where socialization seemed to uniquely affect males and females will be discussed below with an analysis of why these differences may have occurred. The data on which these conclusions are based can be found in Tables 6.2, 6.4, 6.6, and 6.8. These tables indicate the results of a regressed change analysis that show how sex and other variables explain change in orientation from first to last year in medical school.* Table 8.6, based on the regressed change analysis in Chapter 6, shows the proportion of the total sex effect mediated by explanatory variables that predict

---

*Sex and other background variables were measured during the freshman year, whereas other explanatory variables were measured during the senior year. For a discussion of the assumptions underlying the causal sequence of variables in the regression analysis, see Chapter 6.

change in professional orientations over time. Change is examined by using the time-one measures of professional orientation to predict the time-two orientations.[4] By comparing the regression coefficients for sex before and after explanatory variables are added to the equation, we can determine if the sexes change differently over time because of differences on these explanatory variables. Entering each explanatory variable into the equations last further shows which of these variables accounts for differences in orientation change between the sexes. School experience variables such as participation in minority organizations, support of the women's movement, and negative treatment from faculty have been included. For the full list of explanatory variables see the path model in Chapter 6.

The author checked for significant interactions between sex and background attributes (for example, race, school, and social class) and between sex and explanatory variables to explain orientation change; the few significant interactions were dismissed as chance events. Because the sexes changed in the same general pattern at all schools, the three institutions were combined in the data analysis. In other words, differences in educational experiences at the three schools did not seem to significantly affect the sex pattern of change on professional orientations.

If the explanatory variables (for example, negative treatment from faculty and supporting the women's movement) are going to account for differences in the way men and women change in their orientations, then we must first determine whether gender is related to any of these school experiences. As expected, in comparison with men, women were more likely to have experienced negative and insensitive treatment from faculty (.13), perceived that patients were treated in a negative way by physicians (.12), felt that school was difficult in terms of the time pressures (.25), viewed their schooling and career negatively (.13), supported and been familiar with the women's movement (.42), participated in liberal and minority organizations (.39), and disagreed with faculty's and attending physicians' political views concerning medicine (.15)—correlation coefficients between sex and these school experiences are reported in parentheses. These findings are not surprising since medicine has been criticized for its sexist treatment of women and women tend to be more liberal than men. Sex differences on these school experiences did not for the most part insulate women from the socialization process that led to greater conservatism and less interest in patient-need practices. Furthermore, as detailed next, where the sexes did change differently over time on professional values and expectations, these variations were only partially explained by a few of these differences in school experiences.

TABLE 8.6

Proportion of the Total Sex Effect Mediated by Explanatory Variables for Predicting Change in Professional Orientation Measures from Freshman to Senior Year

Professional Orientation Measures	Total Sex Effect	Total Indirect Effect	Total Indirect Divided by Total Sex
Give information to patients	.134	.001	.01
Be critical of doctors	.130	.135	1.04*
Specialty choice pressure exists	.237	.083	.35
Need more women doctors	.194	.105	.54
Bias toward women patients exists	.337	.110	.33
Reduce profession's control	.126	.063	.50
Plan volunteer work	−.141	.033	—*
Plan rural practice	−.110	.017	—*

*Slight suppressor effects.

Note: Tables 6.2, 6.4, 6.6, and 6.8 show the explanatory variables in the equations for each professional orientation measure. Sex is coded so that zero equals male and one equals female.

184

Previously we have seen that from freshman to senior year females were slightly more likely than males to become convinced of the importance of providing health information to patients and of patients being critical of physicians' judgments. Women's greater familiarity with and support of the women's movement explained almost completely their growing critical attitudes toward physicians over time. Table 8.6 shows that the total sex effect is completely explained by explanatory variables. By entering each explanatory variable into the equation last, the researcher noted that familiarity with and support of the women's movement almost completely explained women becoming more critical than men of physicians (see Table 6.2 for the full equation). This finding makes sense because the women's health movement literature is quite critical of relying too heavily on physicians' expertise. On the other hand, Table 8.6 shows that none of the explanatory variables (for example, supporting the women's movement, participating in liberal organizations, or disagreeing with faculty) accounted for why females became more supportive of giving patients health information. Perhaps a more critical attitude about physicians' competence resulted in women advocating the dispersal of health information so that patients can be more involved in health-care decisions. (During senior year, the correlation between giving health information to patients and patients being critical of physicians was .29.) Thus women's more egalitarian attitudes toward the doctor/patient relationship in senior year was only partially a result of their involvement with the women's movement.

As noted in Chapter 7, males and females tended to polarize over time on issues concerning discrimination against women physicians and patients. As freshmen and especially as seniors, females were less likely than males to deny specialty choice pressure on women in medicine, the need for women doctors, and prejudice against women patients. Table 8.6 shows that about one-third to one-half of the polarization between the sexes on issues of sexism in medicine was accounted for by explanatory variables (note the proportions of total indirect over total sex effect). The most important explanatory variable was familiarity with and support of the women's movement. In other words, the ideas of the women's movement helped to maintain women's greater sensitivity to issues of sexism in medicine. Although women were more likely to have participated in liberal and minority organizations and to have experienced negative treatment from faculty, these experiences did not explain the polarization between the sexes on women's issues in medicine. A backlash among the men toward outspoken women may be one reason for this polarization.

On most issues concerning political and economic change in medicine, men and women did not differ in the extent to which they became more conservative. There were two slight exceptions to this trend. Men were slightly more likely than women to become conservative on the issue of government intervention to reduce the profession's control over health care. As shown in Table 8.6, one-half of this difference in change between the sexes was explained by varied experiences in medical school. The most important experience difference was women's greater support of and familiarity with the women's movement.* In addition, women were more likely to decrease their commitment to volunteer work than men. As shown in Table 8.6, this loss was not accounted for by any of the explanatory variables in the model. Lack of time has usually been more of an issue for women because career building coincides with the optimal age for having children. Owing to the added time pressures on women to somehow manage a career and a family, volunteer work, although valued, has probably been seen as less possible. During freshman year, women probably made plans based more on their ideals and thus were just as likely as men to plan volunteer work. In the senior year, women were getting closer to facing career and family commitments and thus their plans probably reflected a more realistic appraisal of their available time. As was shown in Chapter 7, women were expecting to work a lot more than they wanted, which might have contributed to their loss of interest in volunteer work.

Women and men changed fairly uniformly on most expectations concerning physician maldistribution except that women were slightly more likely than men to lose interest in rural practice. As shown in Table 8.6 this difference between men and women in changing their rural practice plans was not accounted for by any school experiences included in the path model. Perhaps women were more likely to view locating in a rural area as difficult because they might be more likely to consider a present or future spouse's professional career when deciding where to settle. Among married seniors, 92 percent of the women had spouses with postgraduate education as compared with 39 percent of the men. Because a rural area might be viewed as a difficult place for two professional people to get work, women might be swayed from this practice choice due to their greater likelihood of

---

*The means for males and females on the index concerning government intervention to reduce the profession's control over health care were the only ones that differed somewhat when considering the subset of respondents who answered both questionnaires (279) as compared to all those who answered the first questionnaire (326). Based on 326 cases at time one and 279 cases at time two, the difference between males and females remained fairly stable over time. Thus the sex difference in change reported here may be an artifact of the sample.

ending up in a two-career family. Fulfilling one's commitment to patient need by practicing in the inner city probably seemed like a more flexible alternative to women. In addition, because women appear more likely than men to desire a highly educated spouse, being in a rural area with few professionals may have seemed more socially limiting for an unmarried woman than for an unmarried man. Thus, women's greater loss of interest in rural practice and in volunteer work probably reflects personal considerations more than differential socialization.*

Involvement with the women's movement did explain some of the differential changes between the sexes on some professional values and expectations over time, particularly those concerning sexism in medicine, confidence in physicians' judgments, and reduction in the profession's control over health care. Participation in liberal and minority organizations, support of the women's movement, and the isolation of women because of such things as negative treatment by faculty of negative role models were not enough to block women's acquisition of more conservative views and of less patient-oriented practice plans. Thus, on many values and expectations, especially those concerning political and economic change and physician maldistribution, socialization seemed to have a similar conservative impact on males and females alike. Orientation differences between the sexes in senior year seemed to be more a function of the selection process into medical school than the socialization process while in school.

SUMMARY

When compared with males, females began medical school somewhat more oriented to humanitarian patient-care values, political and economic change in the profession of medicine, the problems facing women physicians and patients, and inner-city ghetto practice. Personality differences between the sexes accounted for only a few of these sex differences in professional orientations. Women were more interested in humanitarian doctor/patient relationships and inner-city ghetto practice partially because they started school with a greater

---

*Although men were slightly more likely than women to be married, differences on senior-year marital status did not explain any of the students' declining interest in rural practice or women's greater loss of interest relative to men. It appears that a current or expected spouse's career plans may be more important than marital status in dictating students' choice of a practice location.

desire to help people. In the freshman year, women were less conservative on most political and economic change issues and plans,
more aware of sex discrimination, and more interested in inner-city
ghetto practice in part because they were generally more liberal in
political outlook than the men. Because medicine is a somewhat deviant career choice for women, it is not surprising that they begin
school with less traditional values. Although not tested, the author
proposed that women's greater exposure and receptivity to the ideology of the women's movement and their anticipated minority status
may have accounted at least partially for their more liberal professional values upon entrance to medical school. Such contact with the
women's movement seems to have kept them slightly more aware of
sexism in medicine and critical of physicians' expertise through four
years of medical training.

Originally, the author proposed that such factors as the isolation of women in medical school, the women's movement as an alternative ideology, and participation in liberal and minority organizations might prevent medical school from having a conservative influence on women. This appears to be the case only on some issues
related to sex discrimination and to the egalitarian treatment of patients. Women have been more likely than men to remain sensitive
to sexism in medicine and to advocate a critical view toward physicians' judgments due in part to their contact with women's movement ideology. These findings lend only limited support to the hypothesis that professional socialization will differ for the sexes because
of the formation of an alternative reference group for women. By and
large, medical education seems to have a conservative influence on
both men and women.

NOTES

1. For a further explanation concerning the decomposition
of effects, see Duane F. Alwin and Robert M. Hauser, "The Decomposition of Effects in Path Analysis," American Sociological Review
40 (February 1975): 37–47.

2. Daniel H. Funkenstein, Medical Students, Medical Schools
and Society during Five Eras: Factors Affecting the Career Choices
of Physicians 1958–1976 (Cambridge, Mass.: Ballinger, 1978), pp.
73–82; and John Kosa and Robert E. Coker, Jr. , "The Female Physician in Public Health: Conflict and Reconciliation of the Sex and
Professional Roles," in Professional Woman, ed. Athena Theodore
(Cambridge, Mass.: Schenkman, 1971), pp. 195–206.

3. See, for example, Gena Corea, The Hidden Malpractice:
How American Medicine Mistreats Women (New York: Jove Publica-

tions, 1977); and The Boston Women's Health Book Collective, Our Bodies, Ourselves (New York: Simon and Schuster, 1976).

4. For an explanation of regressed change analysis, see Lee J. Cronbach and Lita Furby, "Can We Measure Change—Or Should We?" Psychological Bulletin 69 (1970): 68-80.

9

IMPLICATIONS, CONCLUSIONS, AND POLICY RECOMMENDATIONS

Changes in medical students' professional values and expectations from their first to last year in medical school have been traced in this book. In summarizing these changes, this chapter will address some of the unique achievements of this research. These accomplishments include the demonstration of the feasibility and utility of studying specific professional orientations relevant to health care; the examination of how and why these health-related orientations change, implying the medical school's role in affecting health-care problems; and the focus on the nature, source, and implications of sex differences in professional orientations, a previously neglected topic. Having outlined the problems associated with medical education, this chapter will also present some policy recommendations.

PROFESSIONAL ORIENTATIONS

In the first chapter, previous medical student studies were criticized because of their focus on values that evoke idealistic responses and lack specificity and relevance to health-care problems. In contrast, the present study has examined how students change on specific health-care related values and expectations, particularly those for which physicians have been criticized. The feasibility of reliably measuring specific professional values has been demonstrated, and the results have yielded a more complex picture of medical students than has much past research. For example, this study has shown that most medical students remained committed to the ideal of helping people throughout their training. Yet students became considerably less committed to specific humanitarian plans such as practices in need areas and volunteer work. Therefore, the altruistic picture depicted of medical students previously is much too simplistic. Furthermore, although most students minimize the importance of money and prestige in their career choice, few approved of lowering physicians' incomes and status. By comparing students' idealistic orientations with their views on more pointed issues, this study illustrates a more realistic portrayal of medical students than has most previous research.

One assumption of this research is that these specific professional orientations have implications for health-care delivery and quality. This assumption is based on the author's definition of health-care problems and what constitutes good care. In Chapter 1, the author has shown considerable consensus among critics of the medical profession on aspects of the health-care system in need of improvement or change. There has been some controversy, however, concerning the future shortage of primary-care physicians due to a predicted surplus of all physicians. But with physician overabundance, especially in specialties, it appears less detrimental to the rising cost of health care to have proportionately more primary-care physicians than specialists. [1] Therefore, selecting students interested in primary-care medicine and sustaining their plans is still considered an important goal for medical educators, despite recent predictions. Thus, evidence has been presented that suggests that the professional orientations considered here have relevance for existing health-care problems.

ORIENTATION CHANGE AND IMPLICATIONS

Examining how and why medical students change on specific health-related orientations is another contribution of this study. Many students began medical school with a somewhat liberal and idealistic orientation on many issues concerning the practice and profession of medicine. During training, there was a conservative trend on political and economic professional issues, and students became less committed to practices in geographic and specialty areas of need. These data tend to support the view that professional socialization in medical school results in fairly encompassing attitudinal shifts and the acquisition of traditional professional views. Professional socialization, however, is not a totally homogenizing process whereby students blindly accept all dominant ideologies. Students remained concerned with sexism in medicine and with ways to equalize and humanize doctor/patient interactions, even though many felt that faculty members were not good role models with respect to their treatment of patients.

The present research has not attempted to study the socialization process directly. Instead, experiences associated with medical training were tested for their ability to predict changes in students' professional orientations. Data showed that accepting faculty and attending physicians' views toward the medical profession and toward patients tended to reinforce conservatism, elitism, specialization, and ignorance about sexism. Advocating such alternative ideologies as those connected with the women's movement tended to block conservative, elitist, and sexist trends. In addition, most students described their medical school as a conservative environment that encouraged specialization. Therefore, those who went through training rejecting faculty role models and supporting the women's movement were less likely to succumb to the conservative socialization influence of medical training.

Further evidence linking the change in students' values and expectations to their experience in school results from rejecting other sources of influence. The argument that growing conservatism among medical students is simply a reflection of the change in political liberalism nationally was not substantiated. By and large, becoming more conservative in political outlook did not explain professional orientation change. Other experiences, however, cannot be dismissed as possible sources influencing students' professional orientations. For example, aging, maturing, and personal considerations must have some role in changing students' values and expectations. Thus students may lose interest in primary-care practice not only because medical education discourages it, but because working fewer and more regular hours has become an important consideration. Although medical education has not been the sole influence on students' orientations, it at least appears to be an important factor.

According to secondary socialization theorists, values and norms are internalized during professional training as a result of occupational conditioning and degrading ceremonies.[2] Medical students are supplied new clothes and terminology, expected to work long hours for no pay, and are at the bottom of the medical hierarchy. These rituals help to reduce the relevance of prior experiences, to reshape students' views, and to strengthen the commitment of those who make it (and almost all finish). The analogy is that socialization into a profession is similar in process to induction into the army or a fraternity. Although socialization into medical school is not as pervasive as induction into the army, medical education is a likely source for much orientation change.

As previously stated, one assumption of this research has been that rejecting most of the values and expectations considered here will contribute to problems with the practice of medicine and the availability of health care. Based on this assumption and evidence linking change in professional orientations to medical school experiences, the author concludes that medical education is exacerbating the crisis in health care.

Before going any further with the implications of the findings, we need to evaluate whether medical students' orientations in their senior year are likely to predict subsequent behavior. If medical students' values do not predict their subsequent behavior, then their values may be irrelevant for health-care delivery and quality. The relationship or nonrelationship between attitudes and behavior has been a long-debated controversy among sociologists. Recent studies conclude that the correlations between attitudes and behavior are enhanced if attitudes are reliably measured and conceptually clear.[3] Because most of the orientations measured here are specific and reliable, the author suspects that professional orientations will be linked to behavior. The few studies that examine the impact that values have on actual medical practice indicate some degree of correlation between attitudes and behavior. Seeman and Evans suggest that physicians' support of status differentials between professionals and others is negatively related to the time spent giving psychological support to patients.[4] Davis shows that physicians who emphasize the importance of rapport with clients establish better doctor/patient relationships on one dimension of actual behavior.[5] Physicians' attitudes toward patients were shown not to correlate with other behavioral measures of doctor/patient interactions. Values and expectations are probably only approximations of actual behavior. Responses to specific and reliably measured values, however, are likely to be more informative than vague measures eliciting idealistic orientations. Furthermore, students expectations about future behavior (for example, plans to do rural practice or work for political change) are probably better predictors of future actions than their values, regardless of specificity.

Another stumbling block to assessing the potential impact of students' values on health-care problems is determining the fate of values over time. If trends witnessed during four years of medical school are reversed later in training or practice, then senior-year values may mean little for future behavior. We have seen that medical students tended to become more conservative and less oriented to patient-need practices in medical school. The author suspects that residency training and future practice will further these trends rather than reverse them. Such factors as the long hours of residency training, excessive patient loads, large future incomes, and confrontation of the realities of everyday practice may make these future physicians more conservative and perhaps more elitist and sexist in their treatment of patients. In addition, those who take residency training in such primary-care fields as internal medicine have the option to specialize later in training. The author suspects that many will take that option. Thus the trends started in medical school are expected to continue in residency training and practice.

To summarize, the author makes three assumptions in order to interpret the findings in this study: (1) values and expectations during medical school have implications for behavior, (2) changes in orientation will follow the same conservative trends started in medical school, and (3) the health-care problems enumerated by the author are, in fact, problems. With these assumptions in mind, the implications of the findings for health care, medical education, and the medical profession will be discussed.

Because most senior medical students are fairly conservative on issues concerning political and economic change in medicine, they are not expected to push for major reforms of the medical profession. It is in the interests of these future practitioners not to advocate changes like socialized medicine, a compulsory National Service Corps, and lower financial rewards for physicians. The impetus for reforming the political and economic organization of the profession is therefore not likely to come from physicians as a whole.

Many medical students in North Carolina are choosing primary-care specialties and indicating their commitment to some patient-need areas. Even though the government estimates that overspecialization will continue to be a problem,[6] the recent popularity of primary-care careers has improved specialty maldistribution. The news for geographic maldistribution, however, does not seem as optimistic if North Carolina reflects national trends.[7] Relatively few students plan rural or inner-city ghetto practices, the latter being the most unlikely area for almost all students. Even with an overabundance of physicians, there will very likely be a short supply of practitioners in rural and ghetto areas for some time.

If values have any indications for future behavior, many students may establish humanitarian and egalitarian relationships with patients once they enter practice. This young crop of physicians may be more interested in getting their patients involved with health-care decisions than physicians previously did. They may be less attached to the role of playing God and to the paternalistic values that go along with that role. The rigorous nature of postmedical training, where often there is little time for doctor/patient interactions, may undermine some of these students' best intentions. Furthermore, with few role models demonstrating how to implement humanitarian and egalitarian values, students may fall into more traditional patient-care styles. Patients can also add to the difficulties of providing more egalitarian care because they often expect physicians to play God and often resist taking responsibility for their health. Future doctors may be more egalitarian and humanistic in their treatment of patients, but they will have to overcome many obstacles from other physicians and patients alike.

Seniors have more definite opinions on issues concerning sexism in medicine than they did as freshmen, although these changes have not resulted in an overall increased concern for women's causes. The impetus for changing the prejudicial treatment of women physicians and patients in medical schools and in practice is not likely to come from students as a whole.

We have seen that many students enter school with liberal views concerning political and economic reform in medicine and with career plans that will aid physician distribution. Students' views and career plans became somewhat more conservative and less patient oriented during four years of medical training. Although medical education has not been the sole influence explaining changes in orientations, evidence has shown it to be a contributing factor. Thus, medical educators have been at least somewhat responsible for the undermining of values and plans that may have promoted better health care for many Americans. Admissions committees, on the other hand, have done a somewhat better job in at least recruiting liberal and patient-oriented students.

COMPARING THE SEXES

The third major contribution of this research has been its focus on the neglected topic of women in medicine. By comparing women and men in medical school and by focusing on issues concerning the treatment of women physicians and patients, this research has addressed a new theme among studies of professional socialization.

When compared with males, females started medical school somewhat more oriented to humanitarian patient-care values, political and economic change in medicine, the problems facing women physicians and patients, and inner-city ghetto practice. These differences initially were due partially to women's greater nurturance, lower interest in money, and greater liberalism. The sex difference on liberalism was by far the best explanation for the initial sex variations in professional orientations. Women's greater liberalism was attributed to women's anticipated minority status, to their exposure to the women's movement, and to medicine being a nontraditional career choice for females. Blacks, another minority in medicine, are also more liberal on a variety of issues.

Despite the increased conservatism of all students over time, most initial orientation differences between the sexes persisted and a few new ones emerged. The sex differences that emerged senior year showed women leaving school more oriented to equalizing doctor/patient interactions and men more interested in volunteer work and rural practice. The sexes also appeared to slightly polarize on some questions of sex discrimination, so that the initial sex differences widened on these issues. Women's militancy in medical school on issues of sexism resulted in a conservative backlash among some men.

Originally, the author proposed that such factors as the isolation of women in medical school, the women's movement, and participation in minority organizations might prevent medical school from having a conservative impact on women. This appears to be the case only on some issues pertaining to sex discrimination and to the egalitarian treatment of patients. On political and economic change issues and on location and specialty plans, socialization appeared to have a similar influence on both males and females. Socialization was not, however, a great leveler of attitudinal variation because it was not strong enough to wipe out or reduce most initial sex differences. Thus, the orientation differences between the sexes during senior year seemed to result from the selection process into medical school more than from the socialization process in school.

The implications of these sex differences in professional orientations for medical education, the profession of medicine, and health care are again dependent on how well senior-year values will reflect future actions. Navarro indicates that women physicians will not necessarily be responsive to working women's needs because class loyalties may prove stronger than sex loyalties.[8] In a paper presented at a symposium concerning women physicians, the dean for student affairs at Harvard Medical School suggests that

> given a profession which admits apprentices to the guild
> according to how well they fit its values, it is more likely
> that women doctors will come to be indistinguishable from
> men than that women will revolutionize the profession on
> their own. What worries me is that women will become
> more like men, when the overwhelming need, not only for
> our profession but for society, is for men to become more
> like women.[9]

Evidence presented thus far suggests that socialization, at least in medical school, has not made women indistinguishable from men in terms of their professional values and expectations. Furthermore, women medical students at several schools have been responsible for changing the sexist way that pelvic examinations have been taught at their institutions. Recent leadership conferences organized by women in medicine offer further evidence that women are not yet joining the melting pot of medical conservatism. These conferences have focused on strategies of action to deal with such concerns as the need for women in positions of authority in medicine, improvement of conditions for minority women in medicine, passage of the Equal Rights Amendment, affirmative action in medical school admission policies, improvement in patient care, and establishment of networks between women physicians and women allied-health professionals. The role of women physicians as leaders protecting women's health may become pivotal in light of recent political conservatism, including moves by some politicians to repeal abortion. There is some evidence that women will be an impetus for change in medicine if their greater liberalism, egalitarianism, and concern over sexism translates into action.

Women's greater likelihood of advocating reforms like socialized medicine and lower physician incomes may lead in practice to charging lower fees than men and being more responsive to public needs. Women's lower interest in money does not mean, however, that they will do more volunteer work in free clinics. To the contrary, men plan slightly more hours of volunteer work than women.

Because women have shown greater commitment to humanitarian and nonauthoritarian values, they may develop more egalitarian relationships with their patients marked by better communication and rapport. Some recent studies suggest that women physicians can better empathize and communicate with their patients.[10] Conditions for women patients may also improve if, in addition to being less patronizing in treating patients, women physicians serve as nonsexist role models for other physicians.

Although women may have a liberalizing influence on medicine, the author is not predicting that they will radically alter the structure of the profession. Women continue to be a small minority of the physicians in this country, and their lower-status positions in the profession exclude them from power, influence, and decision-making networks. The need for more than just liberal women physicians to bring about change is echoed in another statement from the dean of student affairs at Harvard Medical School.

> If the attributes traditionally regarded as feminine but better described as humane are to be brought into medicine, men as well as women will have to engage in what promises to be a long struggle to change professional values. I hope women will be willing to take the lead in that struggle but they cannot win it alone.[11]

Hopefully, as they go through residency training, women will not acquire traditional professional views, undermining them as agents for change. As time goes on, however, and medicine becomes a less deviant career choice for women, we may see fewer sex differences among entering freshmen. This may be especially true if the women's movement loses its saliency and if women cease to be minorities in medicine. Because these changes do not appear likely in the near future, women will probably continue to be more liberal, humanitarian, and egalitarian.

POLICY RECOMMENDATIONS

Although students maintained their egalitarian and humanitarian views toward patients, many felt that faculty and attending physicians did not take into account patients' social and psychological needs. Without adequate patient-care role models, students may not know how to implement their humanitarian and egalitarian values once in practice. Physicians teaching medical students need to be reminded that their job is to provide good role models showing how to treat patients as well as how to diagnose illness. In addition, students need to be given feedback and evaluated on how well they interact with patients and not just on how well they learn technical information. Rewarding or reprimanding students for the quality of their relationships with patients should elevate the importance of interpersonal aspects of patient care.

Although the link between physical and psychological health is common knowledge, there are few models in medical school to help students deal effectively with such information. Perhaps a required course on the mind/body link, emphasizing a holistic health perspective, would help balance the overreliance on technical information. Such a course could emphasize research linking stress and disease, patient relaxation techniques to reduce stress and pain, ways to facilitate communication with patients, interaction patterns with patients that maximize the effectiveness of medical treatment, and application of a preventive medical approach. A preventive approach to medical problems would help students focus on the normal body mechanisms for maintaining health rather than on only disease processes. This knowledge could be used in both treating illness and preventing health problems.

Although the delivery and quality of medical care is a politically charged topic, the discussion of such issues as socialized medicine and maldistribution of health services is not considered a legitimate part of medical education. Perhaps medical forums to deal with how existing health-care policies affect the quality, distribution, and cost of care might educate students about possible solutions for eliminating inequality in health services. Students should be exposed to points of view other than those presented by the American Medical Association (AMA) or the drug companies. Medical forums focusing on controversial issues may be one way to stimulate critical thinking.

In recent years, women medical students and physicians appear to have raised their colleagues' consciousness about obvious instances of sex discrimination. Reactions to outspoken women, however, have not always been sympathetic. Women are still underrepresented in positions of leadership within the profession. Recent leadership conferences for women in medicine have addressed some of the problems that women face in a male-dominated profession. Through united action stemming from such conferences, women may realize greater influence in the profession. Thus, the American Medical Women's Association and the AMA should continue to fund women's leadership conferences as well as conferences for racial minority groups in medicine.

Discrimination toward women patients is another problem that needs to be addressed during medical training. The program described previously, whereby medical students are taught how to do a pelvic examination by women in a local women's health group, may prove an effective means for combating discrimination toward women patients. The program trains medical students to do gynecological examinations with greater sensitivity to the social and psychological needs of patients. A preliminary study suggests that this program has improved not only students' examination skills but also has sensitized students to more egalitarian ways to treat women patients. [12] Such innovative teaching programs should be adopted by all medical schools. Because women medical students are more aware of sex discrimination, increasing the proportion of women in medical school may also help improve conditions for both women physicians and patients.

Many medical schools have adopted programs designed to improve the geographic and specialty distribution of physicians. These include family medicine rotations and preceptorship programs where students study with primary-care physicians outside the medical school. The rationale behind these programs is that experiences with primary-care physicians might increase the proportion of students selecting these fields. In addition, because many of the primary-care role models are located in rural areas, the hope is that many students will consider practicing in less populated regions. Studies evaluating the effectiveness of preceptorship programs have generally concluded that these programs do not greatly influence students' choice of a practice location or their specialty plans. [13] These programs tend to reinforce students' prior tendencies more than change their plans. Since these preceptorships are usually taken during students' senior year after career decisions have most likely been made, it is not surprising that these programs seem to have little impact. In addition, if specialists who train students continue to discourage primary-care practice by playing on students' fears of incompetence, it is no surprise that preceptorship programs have failed.

Both the University of North Carolina and Bowman Gray School of Medicine require their senior medical students to take eight weeks of training with primary-care physicians. At Bowman Gray, students train with primary-care physicians in an Area Health Education Center (AHEC), mostly in rural areas. Students at the University of

North Carolina also train with AHEC primary-care physicians, although less emphasis is placed on choosing a rural area. In addition, students at this state school are required to do a family medicine rotation. At the time of this study, Duke University Medical School had no such requirements, consistent with their emphasis on research and specialty practice.* It is not surprising that Duke students started less committed to primary care and were slightly more likely to lose interest in primary-care practices. Lack of experiences with primary-care role models might account for the Duke students' greater tendency toward specialization during training. Therefore, data analyzed here suggest that primary-care preceptorships and family medicine rotations may help maintain students' interest in primary-care practice. These programs might have a greater influence if they were required earlier during training and if faculty attitudes were more consistent with the goals of such programs.

Students at the three medical schools lost interest in rural practice to about the same extent, so preceptorship programs seem to have little effect on location plans. Had these programs been designed to give students more experience with rural medicine as opposed to just primary-care practice, we might have seen a greater effect. Furthermore, because the questionnaires in this study were distributed in the middle of the senior year, many students may have participated in preceptorships after the data were collected. The influence of preceptorships on primary-care and rural plans might have been more dramatic had the questionnaire been distributed later in the senior year.

Other programs designed to encourage primary-care practices in needy locations have been legislated by the federal government. The National Health Service Corps (NHSC) is one such program. Health professional students enlisted in this program are given Public Health Service Scholarships for school in return for service in needy areas after training. Students are committed to one year of service in return for each year of scholarship received. Limited evaluation of this program suggests that it is beginning to increase the number of physicians in rural and inner-city areas. [14] Other legislation presently being considered by Congress would have the federal government pay directly for students' medical education, giving students the option of repaying the loan or serving in a needy area.

---

*Students at all schools had the option of training with primary-care physicians outside the medical school if they wanted further exposure to primary-care medicine, although such training was not required at Duke. Beginning in 1981, Duke will require an eight-week rotation in family medicine.

Students in this proposed program would have more flexibility in how their loan is repaid when compared with students presently entering the NHSC. They would not be bound by a career decision made four years earlier. When students in the present study were asked about a compulsory National Health Service Corps for all medical students, many responded favorably, especially when government remuneration was a consideration. With the rising cost of medical education, it seems likely that a program giving students the option of paying back federal loans with either work in deprived areas or cash would be popular. Whereas the NHSC presently guarantees students' commitment to serve in needy areas, the compulsory payback aspect of this program may limit those choosing to participate. On the other hand, passage of a program giving students more payback options may not succeed in getting enough physicians to practice in needy areas. Both programs clearly have some merits for improving the geographic distribution of physicians and of other health professionals.

Students from rural areas were more likely to begin medical school with plans to practice in rural areas and were considerably more likely to remain committed to this practice choice. Likewise, black students started more interested in inner-city practice and remained more interested in this area. Furthermore, students from working-class and middle-class homes were more likely to express interest in rural and primary-care practices than those more privileged. Therefore, one of the most effective and obvious ways to improve the geographic and specialty distribution of physicians would be to increase the proportion of students presently underrepresented in medicine, that is, blacks, those from rural areas, and those less economically privileged.

To conclude, a variety of approaches should be followed in order to improve geographic and specialty maldistribution of physicians, assuming that these problems continue. These include the following:

1. Requiring rural and primary-care preceptorship programs before students' senior year,

2. Providing more primary-care role models within the medical school (for example, family-medicine programs),

3. Funding more federal programs, which provide financial incentives to medical students to practice in needy areas, and

4. Selecting into medical school a larger proportion of blacks and those from rural areas.

This book has shown that students became less committed to values and plans that are considered by this author to be beneficial for health-care delivery and quality. Medical education, therefore, seems to have a conservative influence on students and appears to

202 / MEN AND WOMEN IN MEDICAL SCHOOL

promote careers that do not meet critical health needs. This trend was partially a result of the conservative and non-primary-care role models encountered in medical training. If future doctors are going to be concerned with many of our present health-care problems, medical schools will have to reexamine their dominant values and career priorities. Selecting more medical students from underrepresented groups, such as women and blacks, may be a beginning.

NOTES

1. Joseph A. Califano, Jr., "The Government-Medical Education Partnership," Journal of Medical Education 54 (January 1979): 19-24.
2. Harold Garfinkel, "Conditions of Successful Degradation Ceremonies," American Journal of Sociology 61 (March 1956): 420-24; and Wilbert Moore, "Occupational Socialization," in Handbook of Socialization Theory and Research, ed. David A. Goslin (Chicago: Rand McNally, 1969), pp. 861-83.
3. Martin Fishbein and Icek Ajven, Understanding Attitudes and Predicting Social Behavior (Englewood, N.J.: Prentice-Hall, 1980).
4. Melvin Seeman and John W. Evans, "Stratification and Hospital Care: 1. The Performance of the Medical Interne," American Sociological Review 26 (February 1961): 67-79.
5. Milton Davis, "Attitudinal and Behavioral Aspects of the Doctor-Patient Relationship as Expressed and Exhibited by Medical Students and Their Mentors," Journal of Medical Education 43 (March 1968): 337-43.
6. Califano, "Government-Medical Education Partnership," pp. 19-24.
7. Ibid.; and Janet M. Cuca, "1978 U.S. Medical School Graduates: Practice Setting Preferences, Other Career Plans, and Personal Characteristics," Journal of Medical Education 55 (May 1980): 465-68.
8. Vincente Navarro, "Women in Health Care," New England Journal of Medicine 292 (February 1975): 398-402.
9. Carola Eisenberg, "Similarities and Differences between Men and Women as Students (Paper presented at the Elizabeth Garrett Symposium, Johns Hopkins University School of Medicine, Baltimore, October 1979), p. 5.
10. George E. Dickinson and Algene A. Pearson, "Sex Differences of Physicians in Relating to Dying Patients," Journal of the American Medical Women's Association 34 (January 1979): 45-47; and Diana Scully, Men Who Control Women's Health: The Miseducation

of Obstetrician-Gynecologists (Boston: Houghton Mifflin, 1980), pp. 93-100.

11. Eisenberg, "Similarities and Differences between Men and Women," p. 6.

12. Jane Leserman and Cynthia S. Luke, "An Evaluation of an Innovative Approach to Teaching the Pelvic Examination to Medical Students" (Presented at the Southern Sociological Society annual meetings, Louisville, Ky., April 1981).

13. Frank A. Hale, Kenneth M. McConnochie, Robert J. Chapman, and Richard D. Whiting, "The Impact of a Required Preceptorship on Senior Medical Students," Journal of Medical Education 54 (May 1979): 396-401; Charles E. Lewis, Rashi Fein, and David Mechanic, A Right to Health: The Problem of Access to Primary Medical Care (New York: John Wiley & Sons, 1976), pp. 61-75; and Bruce Steinwald and Carolynn Steinwald, "The Effect of Preceptorship and Rural Training Programs on Physicians' Practice Location Decisions," Medical Care 13 (March 1975): 219-29.

14. Lewis, Fein, and Mechanic, A Right to Health, pp. 127-43; and Fitzhugh S. M. Mullan, "The National Health Service Corps," Public Health Reports supplement, "The National Health Service Corps in Action," July-August 1979, pp. 2-6.

APPENDIX A

FRESHMAN-YEAR QUESTIONNAIRE

INSTRUCTIONS:

Unless otherwise indicated, questions can be answered by putting a circle around <u>one</u> of the numbers printed next to the answer categories.

1. Name: _____
           (Last)   (First)   (Middle)

2. Date of Birth: _____
           (Month)   (Day)   (Year)

3. Sex:

   1) Male
   2) Female

4. Marital Status:

   1) Single   4) Divorced
   2) Married   5) Widowed
   3) Separated

5. What is your racial background?

   1) White
   2) Black
   3) Other _____
         (please specify)

6. Into which religious group were you born?

   1) Protestant   4) None
   2) Catholic   5) Other _____
   3) Jewish   (please specify)

7. How much importance does religion have in your life?

   1) Very much
   2) Some
   3) A little
   4) None

8. Which of the following best describes the place where you grew up?

   1) A rural area (farm, open country, town under 2,500)
   2) A small city or town less than 50,000
   3) A medium city from 50,000 to 250,000
   4) A suburb of a small or medium city of 2,500-250,000
   5) Within a large city over 250,000
   6) A suburb of a large city of over 250,000
   7) Other _____
       (please specify)

9. At what college or university did you do most of your under-graduate training?_____

10. Is this a public or private school?

    1) Public
    2) Private

11. What is your father's education? (Circle highest level attained.)

    Grade school   High school   College   Postgraduate
    1 2 3 4 5 6 7 8   9 10 11 12   13 14 15 16   17 18 19 20 (and over)

12. What is your mother's education? (Circle highest level attained.)

    Grade school   High school   College   Postgraduate
    1 2 3 4 5 6 7 8   9 10 11 12   13 14 15 16   17 18 19 20 (and over)

13. What is your spouse's education? (Circle highest level attained.)

    Grade school   High school   College   Postgraduate
    1 2 3 4 5 6 7 8   9 10 11 12   13 14 15 16   17 18 19 20 (and over)

    Not applicable (not married)
    21

14. What was your father's occupation during most of his working life?

    _____
    (Please be very specific. Give job title if possible and describe type of work done if not clear from job title.)

15. What kind of business was that in?

    _____

16. Did he work for himself or someone else?

    1) Self
    2) Someone else

17. What was your mother's occupation during most of her working life?

_____
(Please be very specific. Give job title if possible and describe type of work done if not clear from job title.)

18. What kind of business was that in?

_____

19. Did she work for herself or someone else?

1) Self
2) Someone else

20. If married, what is your spouse's present or intended occupation?

_____
(Please be very specific. Give job title if possible and describe type of work done if not clear from job title.) If not married, indicate not applicable. If spouse is working in a temporary occupation indicate his or her intended occupation.

21. Are there any physicians in your family?

1) Yes
2) No (Go to Question 23.)

22. If Yes, please list the physician(s) below, indicating (1) their relationship to you (i.e., father, uncle) and (2) their medical field (i.e., general practice, general pediatrics, pediatric subspecialty, etc.)

Relationship to You   Specific Medical Field
_____
_____
_____

23. Were there any particular physicians other than family who influenced your decision to enter medicine?

1) Yes
2) No (Go to Question 25.)

24. If Yes, please list these physician(s)' specific medical field(s) (i.e., general practice, general pediatrics, pediatric subspecialty, etc.).

                              Specific Medical Field
Physician friend no. 1   _____
Physician friend no. 2   _____

25. At what age did you definitely decide to study medicine?

_____
Years old

26. Before deciding on medicine, did you ever <u>engage</u> in any other occupation or profession?

   1) Yes   If yes, which occupation? _____
   2) No

27. Before deciding on medicine, did you ever <u>seriously consider</u> any other occupation or profession?

   1) Yes   If yes, which field? _____
   2) No

28. How important were the following factors in influencing your choice of medicine as a career?

	Extremely Important	Very Important	Somewhat Important	Not Important
1) The chance to make a real contribution to mankind	1	2	3	4
2) The chance to live a financially secure and prosperous life	1	2	3	4
3) The chance to gain status and prestige with my colleagues and in the community	1	2	3	4
4) It permits me to be creative and original	1	2	3	4
5) It gives me an opportunity to work with people rather than things	1	2	3	4
6) It leaves me relatively free of supervision by others	1	2	3	4
7) Provides me with adventure	1	2	3	4
8) Gives me the opportunity to help others	1	2	3	4
9) Medicine is challenging and intellectually satisfying	1	2	3	4
10) Medicine is (was) seen as a glamorous field	1	2	3	4
11) The desire to do research	1	2	3	4
12) Wide range of options and job possibilities	1	2	3	4
13) The chance to gain respect from others	1	2	3	4
14) Having responsibility	1	2	3	4
15) Using medicine to change society or the medical system	1	2	3	4
16) Other (specify)	1	2	3	4

29. Now go back to the previous question and circle the two most important factors that influenced your career choice.

Primary factor   1 2 3 4 5 6 7 8 9 10 11 12 13 14 15 16
Second factor   1 2 3 4 5 6 7 8 9 10 11 12 13 14 15 16

30. Please indicate whether you agree strongly, agree somewhat, disagree somewhat, or disagree strongly with the following statements. *

		Agree Strongly	Agree Somewhat	Disagree Somewhat	Disagree Strongly
1)	I have little interest in leading others	1	2	3	4
2)	Most community leaders do a better job than I could possibly do	1	2	3	4
3)	I become irritated when I must interrupt my activities to do a favor for someone	1	2	3	4
4)	I would prefer to care for a sick child myself rather than hire a nurse	1	2	3	4
5)	When I see someone who looks confused I usually ask if I can be of any assistance	1	2	3	4
6)	Most people you meet want to get something out of you	1	2	3	4
7)	When two persons are arguing, I often settle the argument for them	1	2	3	4
8)	I dislike people who are always asking me for advice	1	2	3	4
9)	When I am with someone else I do most of the decision making	1	2	3	4
10)	I try to control others rather than permit them to control me	1	2	3	4

*In the following 30 statements, all except nos. 6, 11, 15, 21, and 27 are taken from Douglas N. Jackson, Personality Research Form (Port Huron, Mich.: Research Psychologists Press), form A. Reproduced by permission.

	Agree Strongly	Agree Somewhat	Disagree Somewhat	Disagree Strongly
11) You can't blame people for taking all they can get	1	2	3	4
12) I am usually the first to offer a helping hand when it is needed	1	2	3	4
13) I avoid doing too many favors for people because it would seem as if I were trying to buy friendship	1	2	3	4
14) I feel confident when directing the activities of others	1	2	3	4
15) In this world, it is necessary to judge persons by what they can do for you	1	2	3	4
16) I am not very insistent in an argument	1	2	3	4
17) I really do not pay much attention to people when they talk about their problems	1	2	3	4
18) People like to tell me their troubles because they know that I will do everything I can to help them	1	2	3	4
19) I think it is better to be quiet than assertive	1	2	3	4
20) Seeing an old or helpless person makes me feel that I would like to take care of him	1	2	3	4
21) Most people will give you a hard time if you give them a chance	1	2	3	4
22) I get little satisfaction from serving others	1	2	3	4
23) I seek out positions of authority	1	2	3	4
24) People's tears tend to irritate me more than to arouse my sympathy	1	2	3	4
25) I feel incapable of handling many situations	1	2	3	4
26) I feel most worthwhile when I am helping someone who is disabled	1	2	3	4
27) It's who you know rather than what you know that's important in getting ahead	1	2	3	4
28) When I see a baby, I often ask to hold him	1	2	3	4

	Agree Strongly	Agree Somewhat	Disagree Somewhat	Disagree Strongly
29) I can remember that as a child I tried to take care of anyone who was sick	1	2	3	4
30) If someone is in trouble, I try not to become involved	1	2	3	4

31. This question asks you to think about the kind of physician you <u>will most likely be.</u> Which of the following do you see yourself doing in the future?

	Very Likely	Somewhat Likely	Somewhat Unlikely	Very Unlikely
1) Group practice	1	2	3	4
2) Medical school faculty	1	2	3	4
3) Rural physician	1	2	3	4
4) Primary-care physician* (general practice)	1	2	3	4
5) Inner-city physician taking care of low-income minority groups	1	2	3	4
6) Suburban or urban nonghetto physician	1	2	3	4
7) Physician working in a medium or small city (under 250,000)	1	2	3	4
8) Public health medicine	1	2	3	4
9) Physician working for political and social change in medicine	1	2	3	4
10) Medical laboratory research, full or part-time	1	2	3	4
11) Clinical research, full or part-time	1	2	3	4

32. Please circle the type of location you are most likely to work in. (Circle only one.)

Rural area	1
Medium or small city (under 250,000)	2
Suburb or a large city	3
Large city (nonghetto)	4
Large city (inner-city, ghetto area)	5

*Primary care refers to physicians of first contact offering a relatively full scope of services. For example, family practitioners,

33. Which field do you think you <u>actually</u> will be working in ten years from now? (i.e., family practice, pediatrics, surgery, medicine, psychiatry, pathology) _____

34. On the average, how many hours a week do you <u>want</u> to work when you finish your medical training? _____ hours

35. On the average, how many hours a week do you <u>expect</u> that you will work when you finish your medical training? _____ hours

36. What percentage of your time do you expect to do volunteer work as a physician? (i.e., work in a free clinic, give free care to those who can't pay. Do not include time spent with patients who don't pay their bills or professional courtesy patients.)
   _____ percent   (0 to 100 percent)

37. The thing I expect to enjoy <u>most</u> as a physician is: (circle one)

The challenge and interest of the field	1
The contact with patients	2
The financial and prestige rewards of the profession	3

38. If I <u>had</u> to choose between the following two practices, I'd chose: (circle one)

    A practice in an intellectually stimulating environment but where the need for another physician was not great   1

    A practice in an area with little intellectual stimulation but where a physician was very much needed   2

39. Are you concerned with any issues involving the practice of medicine as it particularly affects <u>women physicians</u>?

    1) Yes
    2) No

    If yes, which issues are you most concerned about? (Please explain.)

    _____
    _____
    _____
    _____

40. Are you concerned with any issues involving the practice of medicine as it particularly affects <u>women patients</u>?

    1) Yes
    2) No

---

general pediatricians, general internists, and gynecologists who do little or no surgery are primary-care physicians.

If Yes, which issues are you most concerned about? (Please explain.)

_____

_____

_____

41. How much anxiety do you feel about starting your medical training?

   1) Very anxious
   2) Somewhat anxious
   3) Not anxious

42. How extensive do you expect your debts to be at the completion of your medical training? $_____(dollar amount)

43. How much money a year do you think a physician working 40 hours a week should make?

Under $15,000	1	$30,001 to $40,000	5
$15,001 to $20,000	2	$40,001 to $50,000	6
$20,001 to $25,000	3	Over $50,000	7
$25,001 to $30,000	4		

44. Do you plan to join the American Medical Association when you become a physician?

Yes	1	No	2

45. Where would you place yourself and each of your parents in terms of a general political outlook?

	Mother	Father	Self
Radical left	1	1	1
Liberal	2	2	2
Middle of the road	3	3	3
Conservative	4	4	4
Radical right	5	5	5
Don't know	6	6	6

46. Would you be in favor of a National Service Corps for physicians in which every physician, male or female, would have to serve one or two years in a medically deprived area in order to obtain a permanent license?

No	1
Yes, only if medical education is paid for by government	2
Yes	3

47. The following statements refer to a wide variety of attitudes concerning the medical profession. After a careful consideration of each item, please indicate one of the following reactions: strongly agree, somewhat agree, neutral, somewhat disagree, or strongly disagree. Remember, there are no right or wrong answers. Please use the neutral category only for issues you have not thought about at all and for which you have no opinion.

	Agree Strongly	Agree Somewhat	Neutral Opinion	Disagree Somewhat	Disagree Strongly
1) It is very important to protect the autonomy of the medical profession against government intervention	1	2	3	4	5
2) Medical training must emphasize learning how to deal with the social and psychological problems of patients as much as learning medical facts	1	2	3	4	5
3) Gynecologists generally treat female patients with respect and concern	1	2	3	4	5
4) The lay public does not have the knowledge required to help organize and plan community health care facilities	1	2	3	4	5
5) As a physician, it will be important to me to have a lot of free time to do other things besides medicine	1	2	3	4	5
6) It is always inappropriate for a physician to make critical remarks to a patient concerning another physician	1	2	3	4	5
7) Patients should have absolute confidence in the judgments of physicians	1	2	3	4	5
8) The medical profession places pressures on women to specialize in certain fields of medicine like pediatrics	1	2	3	4	5

	Agree Strongly	Agree Somewhat	Neutral Opinion	Disagree Somewhat	Disagree Strongly
9) A physician should <u>not</u> become involved in the routine features of patient care that are essentially nurse's work	1	2	3	4	5
10) Medical school and the medical profession are harder for a woman than a man because many students and professors are prejudiced against women	1	2	3	4	5
11) Nurses should have a good deal of latitude in giving information to the patients	1	2	3	4	5
12) Physicians realistically <u>cannot</u> be very empathetic with their patients; it is hard enough to do the technical aspects of their job well	1	2	3	4	5
13) I am opposed to a system of socialized medicine in this country	1	2	3	4	5
14) The medical profession should dictate the location of practicing physicians in order to improve health care distribution	1	2	3	4	5
15) Because physicians undergo long and expensive training, they deserve the income that they make	1	2	3	4	5
16) Review committees should be established by the federal government to insure that physicians do not overcharge for their services	1	2	3	4	5
17) I am strongly committed to locating my practice in an area of the country that needs doctors	1	2	3	4	5

	Agree Strongly	Agree Somewhat	Neutral Opinion	Disagree Somewhat	Disagree Strongly
18) Male physicians tend to treat female patients in a more patronizing way than they treat male patients	1	2	3	4	5
19) Physicians deserve to earn substantially more money than other people in this society	1	2	3	4	5
20) There should be more opportunities for students to attend medical school part-time	1	2	3	4	5
21) We need to change the health care system in this country so that drug companies, insurance companies, and hospitals cannot make profits from health care	1	2	3	4	5
22) I prefer close relationships with patients to large income	1	2	3	4	5
23) Information about diagnosis and treatment should be given to patients so they can better evaluate the physician's competence	1	2	3	4	5
24) I do not plan to practice in a medically deprived area	1	2	3	4	5
25) I feel that the medical profession should keep their control over all aspects of the profession, rather than have government intervention	1	2	3	4	5
26) Prestige distinctions between nurses and physicians should not be reduced	1	2	3	4	5
27) I dislike competition with other people when the stakes are high	1	2	3	4	5

	Agree Strongly	Agree Somewhat	Neutral Opinion	Disagree Somewhat	Disagree Strongly
28) I regard regular and not extremely long working hours as indispensable	1	2	3	4	5
29) I feel a great personal commitment to primary care medicine	1	2	3	4	5
30) It would be damaging to the profession of medicine if half the students admitted to medical schools were women	1	2	3	4	5
31) It is more important for a physician to have extensive knowledge of medical facts than an ability to establish rapport with patients	1	2	3	4	5
32) Women medical students are not discouraged from specializing in certain fields of medicine, like surgery	1	2	3	4	5
33) The patient should be told everything concerning his diagnosis and possible treatment(s)	1	2	3	4	5
34) Generally, I am opposed to government intervention and control in order to solve social problems	1	2	3	4	5
35) Medical school and the medical profession are harder for a women than a man because many patients are prejudiced against women doctors	1	2	3	4	5
36) The medical profession should not set limits on the number of people who can become specialists in over-popular fields	1	2	3	4	5

	Agree Strongly	Agree Somewhat	Neutral Opinion	Disagree Somewhat	Disagree Strongly
37) We definitely need more women physicians in this country	1	2	3	4	5
38) A patient should have access to his or her own medical records	1	2	3	4	5
39) Generally, male physicians are as sensitive as they should be to the needs of female patients	1	2	3	4	5
40) I am strongly committed to choosing a field of medicine where there is a great medical need	1	2	3	4	5
41) As a medical student, I will be very interested in working to decrease the hours a week that interns and residents work	1	2	3	4	5
42) The medical profession would be improved if the public realized the limitations of a doctor's expertise	1	2	3	4	5
43) Gynecologists generally have an accurate view of female sexuality	1	2	3	4	5

APPENDIX B

SENIOR-YEAR QUESTIONNAIRE

INSTRUCTIONS:

Unless otherwise indicated, questions can be answered by putting a circle around <u>one</u> of the numbers printed next to the answer categories.

1. Name: _____
           (Last)   (First)   (Middle)

2. Date of Birth: _____
             (Month)   (Day)   (Year)

3. Sex:

    1) Male
    2) Female

4. Marital Status:

    1) Single   4) Divorced
    2) Married   5) Widowed
    3) Separated

5. If you are married, did you get married during medical school?

    1) Yes   2) No   3) Not applicable

6. Do you have any children?

    1) Yes   2) No

7. What is your racial background?

    1) White
    2) Black
    3) Other _____
        (please specify)

8. Into which religious group were you born?

    1) Protestant   4) None
    2) Catholic   5) Other _____
    3) Jewish   (please specify)

9. How much importance does religion have in your life?

   1) Very much
   2) Some
   3) A little
   4) None

10. Which of the following best describes the place where you grew up?

    1) A rural area (farm, open country, town under 2,500)
    2) A small city or town less than 50,000
    3) A medium city from 50,000 to 250,000
    4) A suburb of a small or medium city of 2,500-250,000
    5) Within a large city over 250,000
    6) A suburb of a large city of over 250,000
    7) Other _____
       (please specify)

11. What is your father's education? (Circle highest level attained.)

    Grade school   High school   College   Postgraduate
    1 2 3 4 5 6 7 8   9 10 11 12   13 14 15 16   17 18 19 20 (and over)

12. What is your mother's education? (Circle highest level attained.)

    Grade school   High school   College   Postgraduate
    1 2 3 4 5 6 7 8   9 10 11 12   13 14 15 16   17 18 19 20 (and over)

13. What is your spouse's education? (Circle highest level attained.)

    Grade school   High school   College   Postgraduate
    1 2 3 4 5 6 7 8   9 10 11 12   13 14 15 16   17 18 19 20 (and over)

    Not applicable (not married)
    21

14. What was your father's occupation during most of his working life?

    _____

    (Please be very specific. Give job title if possible and describe type of work done if not clear from job title.)

15. What kind of business was that in?

    _____

16. Did he work for himself or someone else?

    1) Self   2) Someone else

17. What was your mother's occupation during most of her working life?

_____

(Please be very specific. Give job title if possible and describe type of work done if not clear from job title.)

18. What kind of business was that in?

_____

19. Did she work for herself or someone else?

1) Self   2) Someone else

20. Are there any physicians in your family?

1) Yes   2) No

21. How important are the following factors to you as you think about your career in medicine?

	Extremely Important	Very Important	Somewhat Important	Not Important
1) The chance to make a real contribution to mankind	1	2	3	4
2) The chance to live a financially secure and prosperous life	1	2	3	4
3) The chance to gain status and prestige with my colleagues and in the community	1	2	3	4
4) It permits me to be creative and original	1	2	3	4
5) It gives me an opportunity to work with people rather than things	1	2	3	4
6) It leaves me relatively free of supervision by others	1	2	3	4
7) Gives me the opportunity to help others	1	2	3	4
8) Medicine is challenging and intellectually satisfying	1	2	3	4
9) Medicine is seen as a glamorous field	1	2	3	4
10) The desire to do research	1	2	3	4
11) Wide range of options and job possibilities	1	2	3	4
12) The chance to gain respect from others	1	2	3	4

	Extremely Important	Very Important	Somewhat Important	Not Important
13) Having responsibility	1	2	3	4
14) Using medicine to change society or the medical system	1	2	3	4

22. Please circle the type of location you are most likely to work in. (Circle only one.)

Rural area	1
Medium or small city (under 250,000)	2
Suburb of a large city	3
Large city (nonghetto)	4
Large city (inner-city, ghetto area)	5

23. This question asks you to think about the kind of physician you <u>will most likely be</u>. Which of the following do you see yourself doing in the future?

	Very Likely	Somewhat Likely	Somewhat Unlikely	Very Unlikely
1) Group practice	1	2	3	4
2) Medical school faculty	1	2	3	4
3) Rural physician	1	2	3	4
4) Primary-care physician* (general practice)	1	2	3	4
5) Inner-city physician taking care of low-income minority groups	1	2	3	4
6) Suburban or urban nonghetto physician	1	2	3	4
7) Physician working in a medium or small city (under 250,000)	1	2	3	4
8) Public health medicine	1	2	3	4
9) Physician working for political and social change in medicine	1	2	3	4

---

*Primary care refers to physicians of first contact offering a relatively full scope of services. For example, family practitioners, general pediatricians, general internists, and gynecologists who do little or no surgery are primary-care physicians.

	Very Likely	Somewhat Likely	Somewhat Unlikely	Very Unlikely
10) Medical laboratory research, full or part-time	1	2	3	4
11) Clinical research, full or part-time	1	2	3	4

24. Which field do you think you <u>actually</u> will be working in ten years from now? (i.e., family practice, pediatrics, surgery, internal medicine, psychiatry, pathology) _____

25. On the average, how many hours a week do you <u>want</u> to work when you finish your medical training? _____ hours

26. On the average, how many hours a week do you <u>expect</u> that you will work when you finish your medical training? _____ hours

27. What percentage of your time do you expect to do volunteer work as a physician? (i.e., work in a free clinic, give free care to those who can't pay. Do not include time spent with patients who don't pay their bills or professional courtesy patients.)
_____ percent (0 to 100 percent)

28. The thing I expect to enjoy most as a physician is: (circle one)

The challenge and interest of the field	1
The contact with patients	2
The financial and prestige rewards of the profession	3

29. If I <u>had</u> to choose between the following two practices, I'd choose: (circle one)

A practice in an intellectually stimulating environment but where the need for another physician was not great	1
A practice in an area with little intellectual stimulation but where a physician was very much needed	2

30. Do you look upon your contact with patients while in medical school as: (circle only one)

1) <u>Primarily</u> an opportunity to learn medicine
2) <u>Primarily</u> an opportunity to help patients
3) <u>Equally</u> an opportunity to learn medicine and to help patients

31. Compared with your initial attitude upon entering medical school, do you now feel medical school overall has been

1) More difficult than you expected
2) Less difficult than you expected
3) About the same difficulty as you expected

32. How difficult was it for you to adjust to less free time for leisure and personal interests while in medical school?

    1) Extremely difficult
    2) Moderately difficult
    3) Slightly difficult
    4) Not at all difficult

33. What is your realistic appraisal of how well you have done over-all in your course work compared with other members of your class?

    1) Considerably better than average
    2) Somewhat better than average
    3) About average
    4) Somewhat below average
    5) Considerably below average

34. How extensive do you expect your debts to be at the completion of your medical training? $_____(dollar amount)

35. How much money a year do you think a physician working 40 hours a week should make?

Under $15,000	1	$30,001 to $40,000	5
$15,001 to $20,000	2	$40,001 to $50,000	6
$20,001 to $25,000	3	Over $50,000	7
$25,001 to $30,000	4		

36. Do you plan to join the American Medical Association when you become a physician?

    Yes   1   No   2

37. Where would you place yourself and most of your friends in medical school in terms of general political outlook?

	Self	Most Medical Student Friends
Radical left	1	1
Liberal	2	2
Middle of the road	3	3
Conservative	4	4
Radical right	5	5
Don't know	6	6

38. Would you be in favor of a National Service Corps for physicians in which every physician, male or female, would have to serve one or two years in a medically deprived area in order to obtain a permanent license?

No	1
Yes, only if medical education is paid for by government	2
Yes	3

39. Are <u>most</u> of the students at your school: (circle one)

   1) Highly competitive   3) Somewhat noncompetitive
   2) Somewhat competitive   4) Not at all competitive

40. Overall, is the political atmosphere at your school:

   1) Liberal   2) Middle of the road   3) Conservative

41. With regard to practice and professional issues in medicine, most of the physicians I try to pattern myself after are

   1) Liberal   2) Middle of the road   3) Conservative

42. During your medical training, to what extent have you participated in medical organizations or groups that have a politically liberal orientation (e.g., Issues in Medicine, Student National Medical Association, American Women's Medical Association)?

   1) A great deal   2) Somewhat   3) A little   4) Not at all

43. To what extent have you participated in formal organizations or informal groups (like support groups) that focus on issues affecting such minorities in medicine as women and blacks?

   1) A great deal   2) Somewhat   3) A little   4) Not at all

44. How familiar are you with the literature (like <u>Our Bodies, Ourselves</u>) and issues of the women's health movement?

   1) Very familiar   3) Slightly familiar
   2) Somewhat familiar   4) Not at all familiar

45. The following statements refer to a wide variety of attitudes concerning the medical profession. After a careful consideration of each item, please indicate one of the following reactions: strongly agree, somewhat agree, neutral, somewhat disagree, or strongly disagree. Remember, there are no right or wrong answers. Please use the neutral category <u>only</u> for issues you have not thought about at all and for which you have no opinion.

	Agree Strongly	Agree Somewhat	Neutral Opinion	Disagree Somewhat	Disagree Strongly
1) It is very important to protect the autonomy of the medical profession against government intervention	1	2	3	4	5

	Agree Strongly	Agree Somewhat	Neutral Opinion	Disagree Somewhat	Disagree Strongly
2) Medical training must emphasize learning how to deal with the social and psychological problems of patients as much as learning medical facts	1	2	3	4	5
3) Gynecologists generally treat female patients with respect and concern	1	2	3	4	5
4) Overall, I have greatly enjoyed my medical education	1	2	3	4	5
5) The lay public does not have the knowledge required to help organize and plan community health care facilities	1	2	3	4	5
6) As a physician, it will be important to me to have a lot of free time to do other things besides medicine	1	2	3	4	5
7) It is always inappropriate for a physician to make critical remarks to a patient concerning another physician	1	2	3	4	5
8) Patients should have absolute confidence in the judgments of physicians	1	2	3	4	5
9) The medical profession places pressures on women to specialize in certain fields of medicine like pediatrics	1	2	3	4	5
10) I feel I have sacrificed a great deal to become a physician	1	2	3	4	5
11) A physician should not become involved in the routine features of patient care that are essentially nurse's work	1	2	3	4	5

		Agree Strongly	Agree Somewhat	Neutral Opinion	Disagree Somewhat	Disagree Strongly
12)	Medical school and the medical profession are harder for a woman than a man because many students and professors are prejudiced against women	1	2	3	4	5
13)	Nurses should have a good deal of latitude in giving information to the patients	1	2	3	4	5
14)	Physicians realistically cannot be very empathetic with their patients; it is hard enough to do the technical aspects of their job well	1	2	3	4	5
15)	I am opposed to a system of socialized medicine in this country	1	2	3	4	5
16)	My primary motivation in medical school has been to learn about disease rather than to treat patients	1	2	3	4	5
17)	The medical profession should dictate the location of practicing physicians in order to improve health care distribution	1	2	3	4	5
18)	Because physicians undergo long and expensive training, they deserve the income that they make	1	2	3	4	5
19)	Review committees should be established by the federal government to insure that physicians do not overcharge for their services	1	2	3	4	5
20)	I am strongly committed to locating my practice in an area of the country that needs doctors	1	2	3	4	5

	Agree Strongly	Agree Somewhat	Neutral Opinion	Disagree Somewhat	Disagree Strongly
21) Male physicians tend to treat female patients in a more patronizing way than they treat male patients	1	2	3	4	5
22) Physicians deserve to earn substantially more money than other people in this society	1	2	3	4	5
23) There should be more opportunities for students to attend medical school part-time	1	2	3	4	5
24) I have been pleased with the way attending physicians have met the psychological and social needs of their patients	1	2	3	4	5
25) We need to change the health care system in this country so that drug companies, insurance companies, and hospitals cannot make profits from health care	1	2	3	4	5
26) Information about diagnosis and treatment should be given to patients so they can better evaluate the physician's competence	1	2	3	4	5
27) I do not plan to practice in a medically deprived area	1	2	3	4	5
28) I often have feelings or thoughts that I have chosen the wrong profession	1	2	3	4	5
29) I feel that the medical profession should keep their control over all aspects of the profession, rather than have government intervention	1	2	3	4	5

	Agree Strongly	Agree Somewhat	Neutral Opinion	Disagree Somewhat	Disagree Strongly
30) Prestige distinctions be-tween nurses and physicians should <u>not</u> be reduced	1	2	3	4	5
31) I dislike competition with other people when the stakes are high	1	2	3	4	5
32) I regard regular and not ex-tremely long working hours as indispensable	1	2	3	4	5
33) I feel a great personal com-mitment to primary-care medicine	1	2	3	4	5
34) I have had enough free time during medical school to do the things I wanted	1	2	3	4	5
35) It would be damaging to the profession of medicine if half the students admitted to medical schools were women	1	2	3	4	5
36) It is more important for a physician to have extensive knowledge of medical facts than an ability to establish rapport with patients	1	2	3	4	5
37) Women medical students are <u>not</u> discouraged from specializing in certain fields of medicine, like surgery	1	2	3	4	5
38) The patient should be told everything concerning his diagnosis and possible treatment(s)	1	2	3	4	5
39) Generally, I am opposed to government intervention and control in order to solve social problems	1	2	3	4	5
40) Medical school and the medical profession are					

	Agree Strongly	Agree Somewhat	Neutral Opinion	Disagree Somewhat	Disagree Strongly
harder for a woman than a man because many patients are prejudiced against women doctors	1	2	3	4	5
41) The medical profession should not set limits on the number of people who can become specialists in over-popular fields	1	2	3	4	5
42) We definitely need more women physicians in this country	1	2	3	4	5
43) A patient should have access to his or her own medical records	1	2	3	4	5
44) Generally, male physicians are as sensitive as they should be to the needs of female patients	1	2	3	4	5
45) I am strongly committed to choosing a field of medicine where there is great medical need	1	2	3	4	5
46) My experience in medical school has been predominantly a time of conforming to the values and expectations of medical school faculty	1	2	3	4	5
47) As a medical student, I will be very interested in working to decrease the hours a week that interns and residents work	1	2	3	4	5
48) The medical profession would be improved if the public realized the limitations of a doctor's expertise	1	2	3	4	5
49) Gynecologists generally have an accurate view of female sexualtiy	1	2	3	4	5

46. To what extent do the faculty and housestaff at your school encourage students to choose:

	Greatly Encourage	Somewhat Encourage	Neither En- courage or Discourage	Somewhat Discourage	Greatly Discourage
1) Primary-care practice	1	2	3	4	5
2) Family practice	1	2	3	4	5
3) Specialty practice	1	2	3	4	5
4) Academic medicine and research	1	2	3	4	5

47. Please indicate how stressful each of the following has been for you since entering medical school.

	Not Stressful	Slightly Stressful	Moderately Stressful	Extremely Stressful	Not Applicable
1) The shortage of time	1	2	3	4	
2) Balancing career and personal life	1	2	3	4	
3) Working hard	1	2	3	4	
4) Being a minority student (e.g., woman, black	1	2	3	4	5

48. Not all medical students have the same values upon entering medical school concerning the practice and profession of medicine. To what extent have each of the following groups supported and agreed with your <u>initial</u> ideas about the medical profession?

	Agreed Strongly	Agreed Somewhat	Neither Agreed or Disagreed	Disagreed Somewhat	Disagreed Strongly
1) Female classmates	1	2	3	4	5
2) Male classmates	1	2	3	4	5
3) Your friends	1	2	3	4	5

49. Please indicate one of the following responses for each of the statements below.

	Always	Most of the Time	Some of the Time	Rarely	Never
1) As a medical student I have been treated as a mature and responsible adult by the faculty and attending physicians	1	2	3	4	5
2) Attending physicians have been good role models of how to interact with patients	1	2	3	4	5
3) I have been pleased by the way the teaching faculty has treated me	1	2	3	4	5
4) During medical school I found myself getting angry at how patients were treated by physicians	1	2	3	4	5
5) My experience with the medical faculty and housestaff has been very supportive and encouraging	1	2	3	4	5
6) I have been in agreement with medical school faculty and attending physicians on political issues concerning the profession of medicine	1	2	3	4	5

50. To each of the questions below, please indicate one of the following responses.

	A Great Deal	A Moderate Amount	A Little	Not at All
1) To what extent have the teaching faculty and attending physicians been sensitive to you as a person as well as a medical student?	1	2	3	4
2) To what extent do you support the goals of the women's liberation movement?	1	2	3	4
3) In treating patients at your school, to what extent are the psychological				

	A Great Deal	A Moderate Amount	A Little	Not at All
and social needs of the patient taken into account?	1	2	3	4
4) Have female classmates had a role in changing your attitudes and values concerning the profession and the practice of medicine?	1	2	3	4
5) Have male classmates had a role in changing your attitudes and values concerning the profession and the practice of medicine?	1	2	3	4
6) To what extent have the teaching faculty and attending physicians been racist or sexist?	1	2	3	4

51. Please indicate whether you agree strongly, agree somewhat, disagree somewhat, or disagree strongly with the following statements.

	Agree Strongly	Agree Somewhat	Disagree Somewhat	Disagree Strongly
1) Most people you meet want to get something out of you	1	2	3	4
2) You can't blame people for taking all they can get	1	2	3	4
3) In this world, it is necessary to judge persons by what they can do for you	1	2	3	4
4) Most people will give you a hard time if you give them a chance	1	2	3	4
5) It's who you know rather than what you know that's important in getting ahead	1	2	3	4

52. Did you fill out my questionnaire during your freshman orientation at medical school in 1975?

1) Yes
2) No
3) Not sure

INDEX

ABOUT THE AUTHOR

JANE LESERMAN is presently an Associate Professor of Sociology at North Carolina Central University, Durham, North Carolina. For two years before the fall of 1980 she was a postdoctoral research fellow in the Department of Sociology at the University of North Carolina in Chapel Hill. It was during this time that some of the data reported in this book were collected.

Dr. Leserman's articles in the area of medical sociology have appeared in the Journal of Medical Education and Sex Roles—A Journal of Research. She holds a B.A. and M.A. in sociology from the University of Illinois, Chicago, and a Ph.D. in sociology from Duke University.

Along with her academic interest in medical sociology, Dr. Leserman is actively pursuing ways to improve health care. She is a member of the Women's Health Teaching Group in Durham, North Carolina, an organization aimed at sensitizing medical practitioners to the needs of women patients. She is also currently interested in the effectiveness of relaxation techniques for the treatment of tension-related disorders. Her interests in Tai Chi, dance, and art have helped keep her life well balanced and have aided her spiritual, emotional, and intellectual growth.